FROZEN IN MEMORY

U.S. Navy Medicine
in the
Korean War

Jan K. Herman

ALSO BY JAN K. HERMAN

Battle Station Sick Bay: Navy Medicine in World War II

Carl William Hoodlet, HM2
U.S.S. Haven AH-12
December, 1951 ~ January, 1953

To the
Navy Medical Personnel
of the
"Forgotten War"

Contents

Introduction

When the North Korean People's Army plunged across the 38th Parallel on 25 June 1950, a mere five years had elapsed since the end of World War II. Yet now the finest military force the world had ever known was just a memory. The troops Gen. Douglas MacArthur deployed to Korea to slow the communist advance were undertrained, ill-equipped, and rendered "soft" by occupation duty in Japan. If this was reality with the fighting forces, what was the condition of the medical services charged with caring for these men?

The Navy Medical Department mirrored the sad state of affairs. Whereas the number of naval hospitals around the world had reached eighty-three during World War II, by 1950 this number had decreased to twenty-six, with bed capacity plummeting from 138,000 beds to just under 23,000.

The decrease in Navy medical personnel was just as dramatic. From the end of 1945 to 30 June 1950, the number went from 170,000 to 21,000. The shortage of physicians was so acute that on 9 September 1950, Congress passed Public Law 779, known as the Doctor Draft Law. Physicians would be inducted into the services based on a special priority system. In effect, this law favored those doctors who had gone to medical school during World War II in a program subsidized by the federal government, but who hadn't graduated until after the war ended. These physicians had participated in the Army Specialized Training Program (ASTP) and the Navy Specialized Training Program (V-12). Both programs, inaugurated in 1942, sent qualified enlisted personnel to medical school. They were deferred from military service while attending school, but upon receiving their medical degrees, they had a three-year military obligation.

Nevertheless, with demobilization at the end of 1945, the Army and Navy no longer required these doctors' medical services. Many physicians who had served less than ninety days of active duty were now recalled for the Korean emergency. With the American Medical Association lobbying on their behalf, it was no coincidence that those who had done their duty during World War II were lower down on the priority list. These physicians, who were serving on hospital staffs or beginning practices of their own, felt strongly that they had already done their time in the last war.

Few if any of the new doctor draftees were board-certified or had experience in combat medicine. The most seasoned may have had three years of residency. The irony was that the Navy sent those with the least training and background to Korea. It was not unusual for dermatologists, gynecologists, or pediatricians to become surgeons once they reported to their units. With only a brief surgical background during internship, many of these men found themselves amputating shattered limbs, repairing lacerated kidneys, suturing perforated intestines, debriding frostbitten tissue, and removing bullets and shrapnel from every part of the human body. It was on-the-job training in the extreme. But despite the inexperience and shortages of medical equipment and supplies during the early months of the war, many neophyte doctors were proud of their improvised techniques.

As with all modern wars, the weapons inflicting the damage were high velocity rifles and machine guns, grenades, mortars, artillery, bombs, and mines. At the outset, the North Koreans were well supplied with Soviet small arms, artillery, and tanks. The Chinese communists came to Korea armed not only with previously owned Soviet and Japanese weapons, but with a trove of war booty captured from the recently vanquished armies of Nationalist leader Chiang Kai-shek. Paradoxically, many of the arms were of American manufacture.

Mostly undeveloped and with limited infrastructure, Korea was also a repository of diseases many American doctors had only read about in medical school. Smallpox was endemic, as was typhus, cholera, malaria, tuberculosis, and Japanese B encephalitis. A brutal killer not even found in most medical texts was epidemic hemorrhagic fever. There were thirty cases reported in 1951 and fifty-five cases the following year. With a 10 percent fatality rate, this incurable disease took a heavy toll until the 8th Army established a special hospital near Seoul equipped with several first-generation hemodialysis machines. This treatment reduced the mortality rate to 5 percent. More common maladies—dysentery and other diarrheal diseases caused by polluted water and poor sanitation—continued to tax Navy medical personnel throughout the war.

Despite overwhelming challenges, by the second year of the war, Navy physicians, dentists, Medical Service Corps officers, hospital corpsmen, and dental technicians practiced first-rate medicine and dentistry in Korea at four medical companies, aboard three Navy hospital ships, and in sick bays of vessels offshore. Unlike Army nurses who staffed the Mobile Army Surgical Hospitals (MASHs) in Korea, Navy nurses were assigned only to hospital ships, aeromedical evacuation squadrons, and Naval Hospital Yokosuka in Japan.

Dental care also evolved to suit the needs of the Marines in Korea. Although dentistry was available aboard hospital ships and at the medical company level, dentists and dental technicians also treated patients very close to the fighting. Quonset huts replaced general purpose tents, and 2 1/2-ton 6-by-6 trucks were outfitted as mobile dental facilities and dental laboratory units. It was not unusual for dentists to treat patients within two thousand yards of the front.

What advanced the Korean War brand of medical practice, which was at least one rung up the ladder from the previous war, was the availability of "miracle" antibiotics: Aureomycin, chloramphenicol, Streptomycin, and Terramycin. Penicillin and the sulfas had been used since World War II. Other drugs that advanced the healing art included: the antimalarials, such as chloroquine and primaquine; the sedative sodium pentobarbital (Nembutal); the anticoagulant heparin; and serum albumin and whole blood to treat shock.

During World War II, innovative surgeons experimented with repairing severed blood vessels as they attempted to restore damaged limbs that routinely required amputation. Many "microsurgeons" of the Korean War advanced this art of vascular repair, which restored circulation, and thereby saved many limbs.

Army mobile surgical hospitals and Navy medical companies deployed near the front enabled rapid surgical intervention. Getting the sick and wounded to MASH units or to hospital ships offshore by helicopter, often within an hour after they were wounded, resulted in mortality rates dropping well below those of World War II. In that war, 4.5 percent of the wounded reaching hospitals did not survive. In Korea, the proportion of patients surviving evacuation during the Inchon landing alone reached the remarkably high rate of 99.5 percent!

In the Second World War, amphibious landings in the Pacific required a fleet of hospital ships, which were often employed as ambulances to evacuate the wounded back to hospitals at island bases for more definitive treatment. In Korea, well-staffed and fully supplied hospital ships, as modern as the most advanced back in the States, provided definitive treatment. Less than one year into the war, *Consolation, Haven,* and *Repose* were either on station as base hospitals pierside in Pusan, anchored offshore, or cruising within range of UN operations ashore. Most importantly, all were soon equipped to take patients aboard directly by helicopter. This indispensable team coordination of hospital ship and helicopter revolutionized wartime health care.

When the Korean War began that summer of 1950, who could have predicted how long it would last, how unprepared we were, what kind of enemy we would face, and what kinds of hellish conditions our fighting forces would find themselves in? Navy medicine's ability to adapt quickly and skillfully to crisis had been proven heroically in all theaters during World War II. In Korea, that institution would be tested as never before.

Preface

M*A*S*H the novel, *M**A*S*H the movie, and *M**A*S*H, the ever popular TV show, are synonymous with the Korean War. For better or worse, since the movie was released in 1970 Americans have defined military medicine in Korea by the nightly antics of Hawkeye, Trapper, Colonel Potter, Klinger, Radar, and "Hot Lips" Houlihan. But was it really like that?

"There was nothing funny about Korea," one Navy surgeon told me. He served at a field hospital near the 38th Parallel when the war had settled down to the last two years of stalemate. "My wife and I sat through one episode of *M*A*S*H** and never watched it again. It wasn't like that where I was." Another veteran, an Air Force flight nurse, remarked, *"M*A*S*H* is something I deplore. I know people loved it but I didn't think of it that way. I don't like all the fun and laughter because that wasn't the way it was."

If World War II was the "good war," fought successfully to save Western civilization, Korea has been called the "forgotten war," the dirty little conflict that somehow fell between the cracks, its veterans ignored and their sacrifices overlooked or relegated to obscurity. Indeed, what transpired between 1950 and 1953 is officially referred to as the "Korean Conflict," as if the event required a congressional declaration of war to somehow legitimize the experience of those who fought in it. During a press conference soon after the North Koreans crossed the 38th Parallel, plainspoken Harry Truman answered in the affirmative when a reporter asked him whether the United Nations's move to halt communist aggression could appropriately be called a "police action." Thus was born the term many of his critics hurled back at him when the military situation was going badly.

Whatever the terminology, this first combat between communism and the free world began without a congressional declaration of war, was fought as a UN operation, became bogged down in stalemate, and ended with an armistice and no victory. Nearly thirty-seven thousand Americans died to reaffirm the prewar boundary between the two Koreas along the 38th Parallel.

In the mid-1990s, I wrote *Battle Station Sick Bay: Navy Medicine in World War II*, which chronicled the story of the Navy's medical experience from the viewpoint of those veterans who served in the Navy Medical Department. My goal was to provide the reader an opportunity to appreciate the single-minded purpose to which the ordinary men and women of Navy medicine dedicated themselves in the fight to defeat the twin evils of Nazism and Japanese imperialism.

With the end of fiftieth anniversary World War II commemorations in 1995, I looked ahead to the upcoming fiftieth anniversary of the Korean War in 2000 with the idea of writing another book. There was an entire group of men and women out there who had yet to give voice to their haunting memories. Many were in their seventies; some who had already fought in World War II were older still.

I soon learned why Korea was called the "forgotten war." More than a few veterans I contacted seemed quite puzzled by my inquiries. Many would give the same type of response: "Why do you want to know what happened back then? No one, not even my family, has ever shown much interest."

A seventy-five-year-old former hospital corpsman told me how he had returned home in 1953 after being in combat for nearly a year. A neighbor saw him raking leaves and asked where he had been. When he said Korea, the man shrugged and promptly changed the subject. This vet's observation should not be shocking, since disillusionment with the war appeared shortly after President Truman dispatched troops to a country whose location few Americans could find on a map.

The book was to be a sequel to *Battle Station Sick Bay*, but with one significant difference. In writing about those World War II Navy medical experiences, I confined my interviews only to the caregivers. But now I hoped to provide a more complete perspective by also telling the patients' stories—the Marines and sailors on the receiving end of Navy medicine during the Korean War. How did they incur their injuries? What were their experiences?

I conducted the bulk of the interviews with Navy medicine's practitioners. Neophyte physician Henry Litvin found himself at an obscure place called Chosin Reservoir trying to survive thirty-below-zero temperatures and a ferocious enemy bent on annihilating him and his comrades. Practicing medicine in such an environment was daunting indeed. "Every moment," he recalled, "was like Custer's Last Stand."

A Brooklyn-born dentist, Morton Silver, discovered that it was impossible to practice his profession at Chosin Reservoir where oral health seemed the least of anyone's worries. "It was too serious a thing to worry about dentistry," he pointed out.

Hermes Grillo, a Harvard Medical School graduate, recalled how he ended up at a medical company a few miles from the front operating on scores of mangled young men without the benefit of x-ray equipment and forced to use retractors made from the brass of discarded artillery shells.

Harboring his grief for nearly half a century, another physician, Clifford Roosa, described the day an accidental explosion aboard his ship snuffed out the lives of thirty men in an instant. "We placed them on deck and went through the formality of pronouncing them dead. The whole thing just seemed like a bad movie," he remembered.

Pearce Grove, still fit and looking very much like the sailor youth in his fifty-year-old photo, had been a machinist's mate aboard USS *Consolation*. He excitedly recounted for me the historic first-ever landing of a patient-carrying helicopter aboard a hospital ship. "We knew we were seeing something new, and we thought, 'Oh, my gosh, this is marvelous!' They were coming virtually from the battlefield to the operating room."

Sarah Griffin Chapman, a former Navy nurse who lost a leg in an accident before Korea, told how she fought to be recalled to active duty so she could teach young amputees like herself to walk again. Was the story true, I asked her, that she sometimes roused uncooperative patients by employing the example of her own disability? Indeed, she had. "I'd talk to a patient who was despondent and refused to walk. I was determined that he *was* going to walk. 'I don't know why you want me to do this,' he'd complain. 'You have two legs and don't know how it is. You can't possibly know what I'm going through.' At that point, I'd reach down and knock on my prosthesis. That would generally set them straight."

And then there was the haunting black-and-white photograph from the Bureau of Medicine and Surgery (BUMED) Archives showing a pajama-clad patient scarcely out of his teens and missing his left arm and right leg. Close examination of the casualty tag around his neck revealed that he was a hospital corpsman. Whatever became of him? Did he recover from his wounds and lead a productive life? After a long search, I found Dan Skiles and he related how a North Korean mortar shell changed the rest of his life so long ago.

What about Navy medicine's customers? Not surprisingly, many of my subjects were Marines. Almost without exception, each commented that he owed his life to the care he received. Joe Owen, a former Marine second lieutenant, gravely wounded during the Chosin Reservoir campaign and saved by a hospital corpsman's prompt action, was particularly appreciative. "You'll never see any Marine who won't tell you that the greatest people in the world are his corpsmen."

Retired Marine gunnery sergeant Garrison Gigg, wounded in the first battle to retake Seoul, related his experience. "I'm lying there and can't see with blood all over the place. I thought, 'Well, I'm dead.' Somebody hollered, 'Corpsman!' and he was right there in a matter of seconds dragging me off the street. It wasn't until forty-six years later when I met him again that he told me exactly what happened. All I know is that I owe him what life I have."

A by-product and often unintended consequence of my research was that very kind of emotional reuniting of patient and caregiver that Gigg described. On several occasions, a former patient recalled the name of a doctor, corpsman, or nurse who cared for him. And then, using the Internet's search engines, I located telephone numbers and addresses. These inquiries enabled me not only to track down yet another veteran and obtain the other side of the story, but added a marvelous yet poignant dividend. Patients and caregivers began talking with each other for the first time in nearly half a century! Sarah Griffin Chapman called to report that Dan Skiles, her former patient, had checked in with her over the phone "for a very happy reunion."

Military medical personnel have long been frustrated by a peculiarity of combat medicine. Amidst the fog and chaos of war, doctor, nurse, and corpsman provide their lifesaving services, stabilize their patients, and then lose track of them as the injured move onward through the evacuation chain. Not infrequently, medical personnel remain ignorant of the ultimate outcome. Did that young Marine shot through both lungs recover or not? Coincidentally, I found some answers in my interviews.

Marine sergeant John Fenwick had been nearly torn to pieces by a North Korean machine gun when his early morning patrol collided with a much stronger enemy force. Although Fenwick was hit by enemy bullets, a corpsman dragged him out of the line of fire, applied a battle dressing to stop the bleeding, and then sent him to the rear. During our interview, I asked if he had ever been in touch with that heroic Navy corpsman since the war. "His name was Snowden," he recalled, "but my buddies and I have never been able to find him."

A three-by-five index card in the BUMED Archives bore the name of Glen Snowden, and after a quick search on the Internet I found his phone number in Houston, Texas. Shortly thereafter, Snowden described to me "that very bad day" in 1951. "I patched up Fenwick as best I could and got him aboard a helicopter, but the way he was hit, he never made it. He was just too badly shot up."

I was shocked the ex-corpsman had remained ignorant of the truth all these years. "Mr. Snowden, he did make it. You saved his life!"

"No. No. There's no way he lived with those wounds. I did the best I could for him . . . the best I could."

His voice trailed off, sadly, apologetically, and I found myself repeating that Fenwick was very much alive; I had just talked with him that morning. And then slowly he overcame his disbelief and agreed to call his old comrade and see for himself. I later learned that Snowden's heroism that day cost him an arm.

After conducting more than fifty interviews, I learned that such sacrifice and heroism were commonplace among Navy medicine's Korean War veterans, even though not a single one ever used the word "hero" to describe himself or herself. Getting to know these extraordinary men and women enabled me to answer the question: Was Korea really like *M*A*S*H*? Read their testimony and decide for yourself.

*   *   *

This book is based on the recollections of Korean War veterans derived from oral histories, diaries, letters, and other documents. I conducted the interviews between 2000 and 2002 in person or by phone. Special thanks to Edith Lessenden for permission to use the letters of her late husband and to Mary Waddill for providing copies of her late husband's letters. Thanks also to Milton Heller for allowing me to use Vice Adm. Joel Boone's recollections of the helo deck incident. I am especially indebted to Dr. Billy Penn for his written reminiscences of life as a POW. Cmdr. Nancy Crosby kindly loaned me her priceless collection of Kodachrome slides. These remarkable color images, skillfully taken during her off-duty hours while stationed aboard USS *Haven*, offered me a rare glimpse of the "forgotten war."

A very special thanks to Janice Marie Hores, Assistant Editor of *Navy Medicine*, for her advice, expertise, and the countless hours she devoted to formatting and preparing this book for publication.

The Pusan Perimeter

*I*t was evident from the very beginning that the North Korean invasion on 25 June 1950 had caught the United States by surprise. Almost with monotonous regularity, the highly motivated, well-led, Soviet-equipped enemy dealt the South Koreans and their American "saviors" a series of humiliating defeats. By August, only one part of South Korea had not been overrun. The five-hundred-square-mile area within the so-called Pusan Perimeter, located at the extreme southeast corner of the peninsula, held out against the North Korean army.

Less than a month after North Korean forces crossed the 38th Parallel and President Truman committed U.S. troops to Korea, the 1st Provisional Marine Brigade was hurriedly assembled at Camp Pendleton, California, and shipped overseas. The Brigade consisted of the 5th Marine Regiment reinforced by elements of the 11th Marines, service elements from the 1st Marine Division, air elements from the 1st Marine Wing, Baker Medical Company (later redesignated as Charlie Medical Company and unofficially referred to as Charlie Med) of the 1st Medical Battalion, and a headquarters and supply battalion. Although the Brigade of 6,534 officers and men was trained, equipped, and intended for amphibious warfare, there were still major deficiencies that would have to be overcome before that unit would become an effective fighting force.

The infantry battalion medical sections would go to war with 1 physician and 11 hospital corpsmen per battalion. The total complement of medical personnel would include 14 physicians, 2 dentists, 1 Medical Service Corps officer, 1 Hospital Corps officer, and 154 hospital corpsmen and dental technicians. One clearing and collecting company, which contained two instead of the normal three collecting sections, would be available to provide up-front support for the wounded.

Prior to embarkation, only about 60 percent of the Brigade's hospital corpsmen received some field training, although most of this instruction was inadequate. Of the Brigade's physicians, two came from the 1st Marine Division and had received some training. The others, with the exception of the Brigade Surgeon, Capt. Eugene Hering, had had no training or experience. Indeed, none of the physicians except the Brigade Surgeon had prior combat experience with the Marines in the field.

Because of the late arrival of most of these doctors, the brief time prior to embarkation was required for assigning and outfitting them with field clothing *and equipment. The young medical officers received two lectures on medical operations in the field prior to departure. During their time aboard ship, they would have no further orientation or instructions other than first aid lectures.*

The sobering nature of the situation was illustrated in the Brigade's unofficial medical log kept between 14 July and 26 October 1950. Although the author or authors are unknown, the candid and sometimes irreverent commentary reflects the emotions of skeptical, unprepared neophytes hastily thrown into battle.

14 July 1950:

All hands made last goodbyes to friends and families at 2400, 7-13-50. Went on board USS [*George*] *Clymer* (AP-57) to count noses. Drunk or sober, they're all here and that's phenomenal. Troops, bucolic and alcoholic, stumble on board. Many ships in San Diego harbor render honors as we pass and we return same. Outside the harbor to form convoy and many old hands regretting to see the familiar routine so soon after World War II.

16 July:

Sea becoming rough and many rain squalls. Sick call line increases daily and most are seasickness. Ship's doctor using Dramamine. Turning about 15 knots and making good a little over 13. Ship's crew inoculated. Much discussion in ward room over Korean situation. Question: Are we to be committed to an apparently hopeless situation?

17 July:

We continue inoculation of officers and troops with emphasis on typhus and cholera. Physical exercise started for all hands. To evening school in wardroom; another Korean briefing. It would seem that we are in for a rotten one for the old chivalry of war appears dead and murder walks instead. Considerable discussion about our use of the Geneva cross insignia and arming medical personnel

19 July:

Physical exercise is now a daily chore. More school on Korean customs. Message received that two more Army Divisions have landed in Korea. Maybe the fracas will be over before we get there.

26 July:

The orders received yesterday for Japan canceled today and morale dropped way below par. Instead of Kobi [*sic*], it is to be Pusan at the southeast tip of Korea.

We are, it seems, to be committed in a hurry. Radio news indicates that the Reds are within 100 miles of Pusan at present.

27 July:

We have requested that our personnel be issued carbines and be instructed in their use and care. This request has precipitated quite an involved argument amongst the top brass but [Capt. Eugene] Hering is adamant. Very warm now both at day and night. The ship stinks and the troop spaces are nearly unbearable.

31 July:

First landfall today—an island off the port bow—one of the Shima group. Conducted classes for corpsmen on topside in AM: first aid and shock therapy, reconstitution of plasma, etc. Lt. Mann conducted lecture to corpsmen on .45 [automatic pistol] and M-2 [carbine]. In afternoon, corpsmen and officers fired off fantail for familiarization.

Two days later Clymer *entered Pusan harbor, which was a beehive of activity. The Brigade Commander, Brig. Gen. E. A. Craig, USMC, presented the newcomers with a sobering assessment of what awaited them. The North Koreans were a formidable enemy skilled in infiltration tactics and the employment of agents. They were masters of camouflage, were superior in numbers, and were well led. His orders to his men were brief and to the point.*

"If I asked you gentlemen to be prepared to go into the field prepared for combat 10 days from now, I know you would do it; if I asked you to do the same thing three days from now, I know you would do it; and, if I asked you to disembark your troops, unload your gear, and be prepared to go into the field at 0430 tomorrow morning, I know you can and will do it. Those, gentlemen, are your orders. Good luck and God bless you."

With an almost impossible task before them, the men were up the remainder of that night and the early part of the next day unloading supplies from ships and distributing penicillin, Aureomycin, and chloroquine to infantry battalions. Medical personnel continued inoculating troops before they left their ships, and they made rounds of every ship that had arrived with the convoy to beg, borrow, or steal medical supplies. All night long the docks were a scene of confused activity—supplies coming off ships everywhere and everyway and being piled here and there in helter skelter fashion, ammunition being issued to troops, tanks groaning off to the railhead, trucks roaring around, native coolie gangs sweating under terrific loads, and everything dissolving into the snafu of disembarkation.

Brigade Surgeon Capt. Eugene Hering found the local ranking Army physician to discuss preventive medicine problems in the local area, and there were many. Pusan was clogged not only with refugees escaping the North Korean invaders but with UN troops either garrisoned there or heading for the front. That, in combination with a particularly oppressive Korean summer, threatened an epidemic of malaria, plague, smallpox, cholera, and a host of other contagious diseases. Vector control was an immediate priority, and Dr. Hering arranged to loan the Army one of the Navy's fog generators and a supply of DDT and fuel oil.

It wasn't long before the first casualty arrived at his command post tragically wounded by friendly fire. He and another physician struggled to save the Marine who suffered a gunshot wound of the spine, but the man died shortly after being evacuated to Changwon by ambulance.

The second casualty of the day, a Marine with a gunshot wound to the chest, resulted from an accidental discharge of a .45 pistol, indicating that undertrained troops were clearly more dangerous than the enemy. This fact became even more apparent during a sleepless night caused by trigger-happy engineers [who] fired all night at us, themselves, rocks, anything that moved, etc. At daybreak, they must have loosed at least two thousand rounds. No one dared move, could only dig deeper and cuss.

Later that day, 4 August, Dr. Hering returned from Changwon furious over catching troops filling their canteens at a village well. His shipboard lectures on sanitation had apparently fallen on deaf ears. Inadequate consumption of potable water was already taking its toll, producing a steady crop of heat exhaustion victims.

Life inside the Pusan Perimeter was becoming as unbearable for the newcomers as it had been for the unfortunate refugees. Even though the rainy season was supposedly over, heavy downpours continued. Clouds of mosquitoes and flies multiplied unchecked, and at that point, no one could find supplies of DDT, louse powder, and insect repellent still buried beneath mounds of supplies at Pusan's docks.

There were diversions amid the misery. On the 6th, the log reported: Spent a lonesome half hour in Changwon at 2230—brakes on our jeep locked and there it was. Finally kicked them loose. Returned to CP and small talk with Maggie Higgins and Bob Miller.[1] Maggie had torn her britches in the most interesting place.

Through the middle of August, with the North Koreans threatening the Pusan Perimeter from all sides, casualties continued to be heavy. Helicopters and ambulances brought them in from the nearby front. Friendly fire added to the casualty list, sometimes in freakish ways. On the 8th, outgoing artillery near a command post had unleashed boulders atop a steep hill over an aid station with unfortunate results.

LT(j.g.) Larson, after about 60 hours constant work under worst conditions, has become a casualty. He had been ordered to bed for nite, had bathed in irrigation ditch, was relaxed, and turned in foxhole. At about 1950, a boulder loosened by concussion rolled down the hill and struck him. He suffered a fractured pelvis with possible bladder involvement. Evacuated to Masan by helicopter at 2045.

Correspondent Marguerite Higgins, always where the action was, became a regular during the Pusan operations. Although often appearing as disheveled and unwashed as the troops she was covering, the attractive correspondent always turned heads.

On the 11th, the medical section made an emergency issue of sox, foot powder, and boric acid ointment to Maggie Higgins. Everybody agrees that, as dirty as she is, she'll do. Maggie is somewhat irritated with the Corps, seems that the language employed is a little too uncouth for her. In view of the extent of her own vocabulary, this is remarkable!

By the middle of August, UN forces shifted to the offensive, driving back the North Koreans. Casualties were heavy on both sides. As the front moved farther from Pusan and Masan, medical evacuation became a severe problem. On the 12th, Charlie Med's command post pulled up stakes and moved forward to Kosong.

Very rough trip across rugged mountain range. Quite heavy firefight seen at crossroads—Army show. Sharp lookout kept for snipers along way. No need for adrenalin after that trip. Our slender resources, designed for amphibious warfare, have been stretched and re-stretched so much that a major evacuation problem would be a disaster. The Army continues to support us with three to five ambulances, but the haul from the frontlines to the hospital at Masan is now more than fifty miles of rough, winding road subject to ambush, mortar and sniper fire.

On the 21st, Charlie Med's command post was back south on flats between Changwon and Masan immediately adjacent to an unknown native village. The aroma of rotting corpses permeated the new camp. As always, medical personnel feared the outbreak of disease as troops again ignored preventive medicine discipline.

An extremely exposed position, filthy, crawling with vermin and over-all a heavy fecal odor. Investigation showed many bodies buried in shallow graves around the area. Five discovered in immediate vicinity.... Bodies are in advanced decomposition, graves unmarked, and identification impossible—presumed North or South Koreans. Deodorization attempts made. Took troops little time to discover sundry wells and watering places in nearby village. In this heat, they can hardly be blamed for seeking cool water but the dysentery problem is ever prevalent. Immediate stop order issued and MPs put on water holes. CP area fogged and re-fogged by Mecon unit.

* * *

Snafu Operation
Many of these shortcomings written up in the Brigade log were obvious to the young officers and men who answered the call. Navy physician Lt. Cmdr. Chester Lessenden, a World War II veteran assigned to the Brigade, frankly described the early days of his new assignment.

The Pusan Perimeter was a snafu operation all the way. I was a part of the First Marine "Provisional Brigade," so called because we were organized into two company battalions—instead of three—because there weren't enough Marines to go around. But even so, we had a full complement of service people—most of whom had never worn green before, including me. My first job was to try to make sense out of the terrible medical supply problem. So I was assigned to the Combat Service Group. The First Cavalry Division—Army occupation troops from Japan—had landed across the only beaches, and they were a mess. So the Marine Brigade docked at Pusan, a matter of some derision by the Army. The ships unloaded in a couple of days and sailed away. The infantry companies and most of the support groups, including the medical companies, marched off to the first battle of the Naktong, and I was left behind with about 12 corpsmen and a tangle of medical supplies sitting on the dock, exposed to the weather and pilferers. We were quartered in tents at Pusan University—Pusan U. And you can imagine what the Marines did to the name of our compound.

After a couple of weeks, the Army supply people established a depot with wire enclosures and guards and accepted our supplies. I joined the Fifth Regiment as Regimental Surgeon in time for the second battle of the Naktong—my baptism. MacArthur was committing us piecemeal, but I didn't know that at the time or I'd have been even more scared.

As an intern, I had the usual exposure to trauma, but I soon learned that for the last four years, I had led a cerebral, dignified life. I remember asking the doctor that I was replacing where their blood pressure apparatus was kept.

He told me they didn't have one.

"But for shock?" I asked him.

"You'll know," he answered, and indeed I did.

The first ambulance load of wounded arrived, and there were so many and the injuries so grievous, I couldn't believe it. Where to start? Certainly not by taking a blood pressure. Big scissors to cut away clothing were a lot more important. Gallons of plasma, strong backs to move bodies out of the way, bales of bandages, stacks of splints, and a truck load of litters. These were the tools.

The organization of the aid station was good, under the direction of Chief Petty Officer [Harry E.] Thweatt, but I added one detail the first half hour—that was a body searcher outside the tent. I had turned over a young Marine to find several grenades with the pins pulled, fastened to his clothing with adhesive tape. I wasn't battle-wise, but I knew what a grenade was.

All that day we evacuated wounded to a medical company somewhere behind us—after we had stabilized them—and that night I had my first introduction to an important unit. Graves Registration it was called. But they did not register graves or bury any bodies. They picked up the dead. They were a careful, compassionate crew. They kept the most complete records and treated each body with care and concern. To this day, I don't know where their loads went, but I was grateful for their attention.

I had arrived late in the day. So I had not met the colonel of the regiment or any of the staff officers. I didn't know where we were or what the battle was about. There was dust and noise, tanks and airplanes, trucks and ambulances, and more blood and bones than I had seen in my lifetime. And still the wounded were brought in. I don't remember eating a meal or taking a nap, but I must have.

This operation was bobtailed. We drove to the river, stopped and turned around abruptly and got word to pack up to move. We packed our tools, sent off the rest of the patients, and took our place in the column of vehicles. Our destination was Pusan again. We were in for a lovely surprise—three brand new companies for the Fifth and two brand new regiments with nine companies each. The Brigade had become a Division. We arrived during daylight to a harbor so full of ships you couldn't see the water.

When time would allow, Dr. Lessenden wrote his mother, updating her on his current situation. This letter written 13 August 1950 describes his daily routine in Pusan yet spares her the more distressing details of his profession.

In your August 2 letter you suggested that I probably was in Japan in a hospital since there wasn't room left in Korea for a hospital. Well, we're in Korea for sure and I'm not in a hospital. I'm here living in the dirt, eating from folding mess gear and washing my own socks and skivvies just like the rest of the Marines. I'm with this little service and supply unit, as I've told you, both as group doctor and representative of the brigade surgeon who is several miles from here nearer the front. As I think I've said, the Army is handling our evacuation of wounded and our supplies come from them....

The Koreans are having a hard time getting used to us. Especially with regards [to the] traffic. They wander out in the street without looking, and ignore the horns. The city has put traffic directors at all intersections, but the people don't pay any attention to them. They have their regular police, but they are being augmented by Boy Scouts. Last night on my trip to the hospital we saw a terrible accident. An individual run down by a huge Army truck. The person was dead because they had the body all covered up, and the photographers were still there taking pictures.

One thing they do like, though, is our stuff. We've had to double our sentries and add other security measures because these people can get through our barbed wire and carry off big items. I don't believe they mean us any harm, but they do like our stuff. In fact, we dispose of our garbage by sitting the cans in the street and letting the people help themselves. We'll have to stop that, though, because they won't eat it all, and the scraps they leave are thrown on the street. There are many half-starved curs on the street, though, and they make fair scavengers. But the odor is getting pretty bad over there.

An Army doctor I've met, the public health man, has promised to show me a case of smallpox. I've never seen one, and I plan to bribe the patient with cigarettes to let me take a daily biopsy until he dies or gets well. It will create quite a sensation in New York where I plan to mail the tissue for processing. Most of the dermatologists there have never seen a case either. There's no epidemic here, but it seems there is a case or two hanging around most of the time. Same way with leprosy, although it is not so rare, and they get one every once in a while at the Skin and Cancer clinic.

* * *

Culture Shock

August also saw the arrival in Korea of the first U.S. Navy hospital ship, USS Consolation *(AH-15), on the 16th. Even as her lines were made fast to Pier 1, the enormous concrete structure hummed with activity. The ship's medical staff immediately made arrangements with the Army Logistic Command for handling patients, records, and procurement of blood and other supplies. The impending arrival of scores of wounded required immediate streamlining of normal procedures. Patients, traditionally admitted at the Medical Officer of the Day's office, were instead triaged by teams of physicians, dentists, and Medical Service Corps officers as they were unloaded from ambulances on the dock. There they were assigned to upper or lower bunks in various wards by numbered and colored tags. Because most of the casualties were surgical*

*cases, both the chief of medicine and the neuropsychiatrist supervised the
sorting, leaving the surgeons free to work in the ship's operating rooms. Line
officers off watch and men from the deck, engineering, and supply divisions
helped in handling patients.*

*One of those crewmembers, Pearce Grove, had joined the Navy on the eve of the
Korean War. The 19-year-old youth found much to impress him. There was the huge
white vessel itself. "I was just amazed! I never dreamed of such a huge hospital
floating in the water." And then there was his encounter with Korea, specifically
Pusan, a city under siege—jam-packed with refugees, defeated and dispirited
South Korean soldiers, and a smattering of UN troops thrown into the breach.*

It was early August. The [Pusan] Perimeter had been pushed back so close to
Pusan that you could see and hear all the gunfire. The real question when we got
there was holding that little piece of land.

We came immediately to a pier, a huge pier. When we came to the dock, there
was a whole row of Korean women sweeping the large pier below us. One of
the women dropped down to her knees and another lady nearby left her place in
line, came over and delivered a baby. The woman then wrapped the infant, tied
it on the mother's back, and the two women went right back in their place and
continued sweeping! This was no more than maybe two or three minutes; it was
very quick. Of course, a teenager, I was mortified but soon learned that many
things in Korea had continued for centuries with little change. Here you had this
ultra-modern hospital ship and a baby being delivered on the dock without any
care.

We stayed and, of course, treated people immediately when they came or were
delivered to the dock. They were mostly American military, but we also treated
Korean military. We all pitched in carrying them aboard. We carried hundreds
aboard the first day. I think I saw the first wounded Korean military man die aboard
ship. That was quite a shock for a young sailor of nineteen.

I also saw men on the operating tables with their entire stomachs hanging
out. I saw them put back together, sewn up, and they lived. I was assured
that these men survived. It was incredible. It appeared at that time that our
hospital staff were miracle workers, putting people back together. Many you
thought would die were soon on the decks to get fresh air, sunshine, and
exercise. I talked to hundreds while they were recovering. We were just awed
by the complexity of the medical facilities of the ship, and the ability to do
what they did.

Pusan was nearly overrun with dirty, wide streets. I was there many times
but this first time I saw more of the traditional elderly men wearing ancient
Korean hats. They were made of a special bamboo or something. They were

lovely and very intricate. You saw a lot of very traditional dress on both men and women. But everything was dirty. There was nothing to keep down all of the dust and dirt from the streets. There were soldiers and military machines coming and going all the time. And so it was confusion with everyone rushing around.

It was at this time where I first saw a lot of the Korean kids attaching themselves to army units. They would clean and wash soldiers' clothes. The soldiers would give them money and, occasionally, cigarettes and chocolates. They, especially the boys, became an informal part of the military service units.

There was a sense of impending doom at that time, August of 1950. When we first arrived it was very ominous. Then the tide began to turn and we began pushing the North Koreans back, not very long before the time of the Inchon invasion.

I should mention that well before we went to Inchon I was sent ashore on patrol duty. In interacting with the people ashore, I learned a lot of things for the first time. For example, as the trains were leaving Pusan and heading toward the frontlines, American soldiers would drop off the train all along the way and filter back into Pusan. The MPs I worked with on shore patrol had lots of stories. Their primary job at Pusan was rounding up the stragglers, putting them back on the trains to go back up to the frontlines. They'd put them back aboard and many would begin dropping off again all along the way. Then they would put them aboard again. I never heard that any were shot for desertion, even though lots of them were constantly jumping off the slow moving trains and coming back into town.

Notes
[1]Marguerite Higgins was a reporter for the *New York Herald Tribune*. Robert C. Miller worked for United Press.

From Inchon to Seoul

*O*n paper, what would turn out to be Gen. Douglas MacArthur's greatest triumph
was anything but a certainty. The troops, who had rushed to Pusan in early
August and had already been bloodied along the Naktong River, were about to be
reinforced by Marines from the States. On 13 September 1950, two days before the
scheduled Inchon landing, the 1st Provisional Marine Brigade officially dissolved
as it became part of the 1st Marine Division.

*The Division was hastily reinforced with physicians and hospital corpsmen
drawn from naval hospitals and other assignments, including the Reserve. Many
of the new men, as with their Provisional Brigade predecessors, had received little
training, and some had received none at all. Now all of them were about to embark
upon the biggest and most complicated amphibious operation since World War II.
Each would see Inchon and its aftermath from his own unique perspective.*

Hospital Corpsman Bill Davis, 1st. Battalion, 7th Marines

About the time the Marines and the Army were in the Pusan Perimeter, they
were especially looking for corpsmen. We flew out to San Diego and got a bus to
Camp Pendleton. We went to Tent Camp No. 2, up near the northern end of Camp
Pendleton and the San Clemente gate.

When we got there, they were forming the 7th Regiment of the 1st Marine
Division. Sixty percent of that regiment turned out to be Reserves, units from
different cities. Some of them were seventeen years old; some were thirty years
old and World War II veterans. Some didn't even have boot camp. None had any
shots or health records. None of them had dog tags. For some reason, in addition
to giving shots and making up health records, the corpsman's job was making dog
tags. This was something I never could understand.

We were there for two weeks and never did go to Field Medical Service School.
We went to the rifle range three times. Two of the times we pulled targets. The
third time it was dusk and we couldn't even see the targets. So that was my military
training. The next day they let us go out in the dark and throw one hand grenade.
I never saw a doctor while we were there to give us any kind of field medicine

education. Then we went down on September 1st and boarded a ship, the USS *Okanogan* (APA-220) at San Diego and headed for Japan.

The plan was that we would go up in the mountains of Japan and get cold weather training. In the interim, on the way over there, Douglas MacArthur decided to land at Inchon so we never got off the ship and never got any further training. On the way over on that ship they would take us corpsmen back to the fantail and throw great big gold-colored coffee cans over the side forward, and we would lay on the deck and shoot at those with carbines they issued to us.

We had a doctor who attempted to give us some field medicine training, except he was a lieutenant (j.g.) and he had been drafted into the Navy and was out of medical school for eight months. He didn't know a thing about field medicine. In fact, he joined us on the pier at San Diego. He hadn't even gone to Camp Pendleton. That was it.

We had a machine at the dispensary when we were doing the dog tags. By the time we were ready to leave, we hadn't finished making dog tags for everybody in the battalion so we got aboard ship and the shipfitter cut out aluminum squares and gave us a die set and a hammer. So we made two dog tags for each person who didn't have them from these squares of aluminum with rough edges and a hole punched in them. And we did it with one die at a time.

We were all in a troop compartment, which was eight bunks high. I had the top bunk because I was smaller than all those ugly Marines. I was lying right under one of the pipes surrounded by asbestos. If you jumped off to get down, you landed either on a jeep or a howitzer, or something they had tied on the deck below. It was pleasant weather so they let us stay up on deck at night. I was up on deck all the time anyway because that's where I was making those crazy dog togs.

Right before we got to Kobe, we had to give everyone encephalitis shots for Japanese brain fever. And that afternoon we caught the tail end of a typhoon. The ship was rocking left and right. Four thousand people were throwing up all over the place. That encephalitis shot will make you dizzy and sick if you're on dry land, but it really did a number on everybody on that ship.

I went ashore on a landing craft that could carry two tanks. We had to climb down the side on cargo nets which I had never done before. A Marine told me to hold on to the verticals and put my feet on the horizontals. It was fairly simple.

Hospital Corpsman Donald Lyon, 2nd Battalion, 5th Marines

The landing wasn't that highly contested. They had taken Wolmi-do Island the day before and so there wasn't that much resistance. But once we landed there was some intermittent fire.

We had to climb up a ladder because of the sea wall. Along the beach was a trench the North Koreans had used, and we ended up in there. Suddenly we heard someone yell "Corpsman!" so we went out on the beach and treated him. We had just finished and were lying in the sand starting to get up when we were hit with a grenade. [My partner] got most of the shrapnel; I got a little but most of the concussion. I helped him back to an LST [Landing Ship, Tank] that had landed. The corpsman there treated both of us and we stayed aboard until the next morning.

I got it on the right side of the arm and the head, and he got it all on his left side. He ended up going back to Japan. The next day we were transferred to the USS *Consolation*. The LST went back out into the harbor and I think they transferred us to the hospital ship by what they call a bosun's chair. That was on the 16th.

Lt. Robert J. Fleischaker, MC, 3rd Battalion, 1st Marines

We went aboard LSTs in Kobe on the 9th of September and sailed the following morning. We then sailed around the Korean peninsula and got caught in the tail end of a typhoon. There was a lot of rocking in those flat-bottomed ships. The Fifth Marines were the main assault force because they had had more experience. They were given Red Beach.

There was a tremendous tide variation at Inchon, which is one of the few places in the world that has this. It amounted to about thirty feet. At low tide there were about three miles of mud flats offshore which prevented anybody from going in or out from the beach. There were only two times a day which at that time of the year happened to be just after dawn and late afternoon when boats could get in or out. When we went ashore in the afternoon, we knew we wouldn't be able to evacuate any casualties until the following morning. Nor would we be able to have any further reinforcements. When we went ashore, there was very little resistance although there were some wounded.

The first time I had gotten into one of the landing craft was when we did it for real; there wasn't any rehearsal. It wasn't like Normandy. We did it for real the first time. I didn't have to go down a cargo net. We went down into the hold of the LST and climbed into amphibious tractors.

We could see where the cruisers were shelling the place before we got in. The industrial area where we went in was just a bunch of old abandoned factories and some old naval barracks the Japanese had built. It was fairly empty when we went ashore. There was some small arms fire and a few people were hit on the beach.

We took care of some casualties that night in one of these barracks. The windows had been shattered in some previous action so we put up blankets to black out the place, and we used flashlights for light.

For medical supplies we just had the first aid kits we went ashore with, what we had on our backs. The kits contained battle dressings, sulfa powder. We had little instrument kits with hemostats and scissors.

I'm not sure we had plasma that first night, but we did subsequently when they got all our gear ashore and things got organized. We had the old plasma units that consisted of two bottles. One of them had the dried plasma, the other distilled water. You mixed the two together, shook it up, and tried to get it all into solution. There was a double-ended needle going through a rubber-capped stopper. You poked it into the one containing the water and then into the bottle with the plasma. The vacuum would draw the water into the bottle containing the plasma. In the field it was used that way. The needles were capped to keep them sterile, and there was also tubing. You injected the needle into a patient, hung up the bottle, and administered the intravenous plasma.

Lt. Cmdr. Chester M. Lessenden Jr., MC, Regimental Surgeon, 5th Marines

Planning had been under way for the landing at Inchon for a week or so while we held our finger in the dike, and the mimeograph machines had gone mad. Someone gave me a stack of papers the size of a San Francisco phone book—the order of battle. There was also a map of a place called Inchon. Meetings were interminable while roles were sorted out. I was assigned a nook on a clean, comfortable ship, and I met a person who was to become an important man in my life and one who has remained a friend, Lt. Col. Ray Murray, now Major General. Lt. Col. Murray was CO of the Fifth. Despite the pressures on him, he took time to explain my duties and to tell me what would be expected of me in this most complicated of military maneuvers, an amphibious landing.

I learned that Inchon had huge tides—25 feet or more between ebb and flood during certain days of the month. This meant there was a mile or more of mud flats exposed during ebb when nothing could cross, while the water washed the seawall at flood. Our landing had to be within a two-day period of the month. There would be enough water to float the assault troops, and me, for about two hours, following which it would be eight or ten hours before we had contact with our mothering fleet again. During that time we would be on our own without any hope of reinforcements, but worse yet, there would be no medical evacuation for this period. It also meant that lots of medical gear had to go ashore with us since all casualties would have to be handled with what we had with us. Everybody had a burden. I and a dental corpsman named Howard carried 48 blankets in a waterproof pack. We were to carry this up the scaling ladders.

Somehow I forced myself over the side of the ship, down the landing net, and into the Higgins boat with the blankets. We idled forward to the departure line where some guy with a flag was stationed in a boat, holding the assault boats in line, until we were all assembled, then waved his flag and away we went. Since time was so short, all the assault waves were compressed, one after the other, so that we were landed on top of one of the infantry companies. The coxswain of the boat was hit just as we bumped the sea wall. Howard stopped to help him, and I carried the blankets up the scaling ladder, over the sea wall, and into a trench myself.

Prior to the landing, a good friend and I had gotten hold of some Aureomycin, a brand new drug, and we had proceeded to try to sterilize our bowels by taking this stuff because there wouldn't be anybody to fix us if we got a perforated viscus. We had succeeded beyond our wildest dreams. Aureomycin isn't used much anymore, partly because it produces diarrhea.

I later learned that there was not much opposition. There seemed a lot to me. But I do know that we were not called upon to handle very many wounded. We were set up and operating in minutes. Space on the beach was at a premium, but Chief Thweatt had a spot staked out in some kind of shed and we gathered there. A hundred yards down the beach, an LST was against the sea wall and was discharging vehicles. Some guy from the top of the LST was firing at the tops of the surrounding hills when somebody from the beach hollered to him that there were Marines up there. This gave me comfort to know that the battle lines were that far away.

Lt.(j.g.) Henry Litvin, MC, 2nd Battalion, 5th Marines

I drove up to Newport, Rhode Island, to start my Navy career in mid-July. I had my white uniforms, I had a tux, and I was all set for a great season. I was there three days when someone handed me orders that read FMF.

I had no clue what FMF meant and I asked a fellow what this FMF was.

"Fleet Marine Force."

I said, "You have the wrong person. I'm in the Navy."

He then explained to me that the Marine Corps used Navy doctors. I assumed that since I was going to the Fleet Marine Force, I would probably wind up in Korea. When I got there and landed at Inchon, I hadn't had one minute of indoctrination, boot camp, or anything resembling training.

I flew out to Pendleton and that was kind of chaotic. Then I was sent to the amtracs [amphibious tractors] battalion and we were loaded aboard ship. When we got to Kobe after a two- or three-week trip, a lot of young officers reassured me, "Not to worry, doc. You're going to be with an amtrac battalion and you won't be with the infantry." So I took some comfort in that. But as soon as we got to Kobe I was transferred to an infantry battalion. I was a lieutenant (j.g.). "Doc" was my title.

The first time I remember being together with the 2nd Battalion, 5th Marines, was at Inchon during the initial assault. On 3 September 1950 in the middle of Typhoon Jane, 20 corpsmen and I had reported to Lt. Uel Peters, CO of Fox

Company, aboard ship in Kobe. His company would give Col. [Harold] Roise's 2nd Battalion its third rifle company. We would join up with the other companies for the landing at Inchon.

When we got to Inchon some of the guys helped me put a pack on, which I could barely carry because I was not in good shape. I had been a busy intern who hadn't done much about exercise or any kind of conditioning. I had a pack on my back for the first time on the 15th of September.

We were not briefed at all. I heard scuttlebutt. We were going to land somewhere. And then while I was standing there on deck I saw planes strafing the beach and vessels bombarding the beach. There was a war going on and I figured I was in trouble. I wondered how one avoided getting shot. I'm a doc and what am I supposed to do? It was 5:40 in the afternoon. There was a light rain and you could smell the cordite.[1]

When I got to the edge of the ship, I saw a cargo net for the first time in my life. And I saw that little landing craft way down. I quickly ended up with my feet in one rung, my hands in the very next rung, and the rest of me hanging like a sack of potatoes. I was on my way down but had managed to get one foot at one level and my hands on the next level. Some Marine climbing down next to me guided me and I made it down.

I carried some medical equipment, but mostly clothes and blankets, shelter halves, and an entrenching tool, stuff I'd never seen before. I was handed a carbine several hours before we climbed down the cargo net. I asked for a .45 instead thinking it would be easier to carry.

The next thing I knew we were hitting Red Beach. There was a 10-foot seawall. The front of the landing craft opened up and, of course, I saw these young kids running and climbing up that wall, so I figured I had better do the same thing. There was a hell of a racket—shells blowing up all over the place, ships firing overhead. I couldn't climb up the wall; I didn't have the strength. And then the next wave of Marines came in and I got thrown over it. I was in the eighth wave at Red Beach and was helped over the sea-wall by Marines from the ninth wave.

So we ended up on the beach being fired upon by the North Koreans and also from our own LSTs. Their 20mm cannons were shooting at Korean positions but their fire was dropping into where we were.

I remember very vividly my first casualty. Actually that first casualty I couldn't treat. He was a sergeant who stood up with a red bandanna and tried to wave off our LST's 20mm cannon fire. He was cut in half. Later on, we were in a little store we were using for an aid station. They brought a guy in with a gaping thigh wound. He had a tourniquet on below it—below the wound. He was completely bled out—white. That was the second casualty I saw, and I couldn't do anything for him.

When you see the first wounded guy, you just do what comes naturally. The item we used most were battle dressings. They looked like giant Band-Aids but instead of adhesive, you just wrapped them around the wound and tied them. They were very handy.

There were two chief hospital corpsmen named Nunn and Hill who I tried to follow and watch because I heard they had been in the Pacific. I figured they had some experience and knew what to do.

We were pinned down for maybe an hour or two. When I saw guys getting up and moving, I got up and moved with them. I didn't like the idea of being left alone.

* * *

The landing at Inchon, was not unopposed, but troops met little resistance and casualties were relatively light. Lying offshore in water deep enough to escape Inchon's notorious tides and enemy fire was USS Consolation. *The LSTs and transports that had brought the troops also stood by to augment the hospital ship's treatment of the wounded. Evacuation skills honed during World War II were in evidence everywhere, but very much hindered by twice daily low water.*

Even before resistance in the shattered city was completely broken, Marines and Army troops were on their way to liberate the Korean capital. As they neared the strategically important Kimpo Airport, resistance stiffened and casualties mounted. Taking Seoul would not be a cakewalk.

Rear Adm. Joel Boone, MC, USN

After a good night's sleep on the USS *Rochester*, provision was made for me to go ashore at Inchon. At "B" Beach I was greeted by Capt. Eugene R. Hering, MC, senior medical officer with the Marines at Inchon. He was a very able young man, most enthusiastic about field duty. He did a superb job in Korea.

Hering was a tremendously energetic fellow. He guided [my aide, Cmdr. Allen] Bigelow and me to see the destruction of the city; it was a shambles. Then he took Bigelow and me in a jeep out into the countryside. There were many dead Koreans alongside the Inchon-Seoul Highway. From higher ground we could see the valley toward Seoul. We had not gone very far when Hering thought we should turn back as we were in range of enemy fire.

There were many refugees on the road. Oxen and human beings were the beasts of burden. The scene reminded me of my days in France during World War I. I saw long lines of refugees carrying what few possessions they could put together in great haste to travel over many miles of terrain, trying to seek safety and protection in the rear of our military forces. The populace was doing the same in Korea, as in France. Appearance of native people were in marked contrast one to the other.

I saw a lot of devastation, many burning dwellings and North Korea tanks set afire by napalm and by the fire of our ships, of the Marine Corps field guns and, obviously, also from rifles when there were close-order engagements. When I first saw napalm destroying a tank or a piece of property or an individual, I was stunned. The ejectors could fire the napalm at a considerable distance. They really created havoc in materiel and human destruction. Napalm, which I had never seen before, ejected as a powerful flame and which seared tanks and caused destruction to anything and anybody in its path.

On this first exploration ashore, I got a very clear idea of the battle raging. It was obvious that United States forces were making very rapid progress throughout the city and well out into the countryside. They were directing their approach toward Kimpo Korean Airfield, which was the largest Korean airfield that they had, and with two good runways. It was a prize which the Americans wished to obtain as rapidly as possible.

Hospital Corpsman Bill Davis, Co. B, 1st. Battalion, 7th Marines

We landed at Inchon on September 21, six days after the 5th and the 1st Marines had landed there, and proceeded to move toward Seoul.

For equipment we ended up with all the stuff that was left over from World War II, some of which should have been burned or destroyed. The mortars wouldn't go far enough or the rifles weren't firing properly because they'd been sitting in storage somewhere. A lot of the medical gear was left over. We had a bag from World War II. It was called a Unit 1. It was a fairly good-sized bag to carry, and it was quite heavy because it was filled with bandages and a surgical kit with a bandage scissors.

In addition to that you had to carry a carbine which only got in the way. I didn't carry a sidearm at that time because they had issued us carbines. After we had been there for three weeks, they called all those carbines back because their range was so short that the people who had them—sergeants and officers—tended to be shooting too close to the troops who were in front of them. So they took those back and gave us M1s. Well, the damn M1 felt like it weighed more than I did. At that time I probably weighed about 105 pounds. Two or three days after trying to do my job with that thing, I gave it to the company gunnery sergeant and told him that I couldn't carry a rifle and do my job. He asked me if I wanted a carbine and I told him I really didn't want anything. Four days later I had a casualty—a machine gunner—who carried a .45. He said, "Doc, do you want this .45?" It was in a blond leather holster. I thought even John Wayne would put one of these on. So I strapped on the .45 and carried it until we got to the 38th Parallel.

So I got the pistol in September and never took it out of the holster until we were surrounded by the Chinese in late October. When I fired it, about two pounds of dirt came out of the barrel. The platoon sergeant said, "Doc, put that thing away. You throw grenades; I'll fire weapons." But that's the only time I ever fired it and it's lucky it didn't blow up in my face.

It's not very far from Inchon to Seoul but we moved through rice paddies, and on the road on up there we saw a lot of tanks and trucks on fire, but we didn't see that many casualties.

However, I had my first casualty between Inchon and Seoul. The guy was shot through the upper part of his leg, around the femur. And the bullet went through his gonads. That's a bandage job that will defy any ingenuity. But I did it with a couple of bandages. I took off my field jacket and put it under him because we were in a rice paddy. He asked me not to leave him and I didn't.

I stayed with him and it began to get dark. The North Koreans then began firing green flares which gave me enough light to see a group of people walking on the dike surrounding the rice paddy. I knew they were Americans because I could see the silhouette of the radio on someone's back. I hollered out and pretty soon they stopped and four or five of them spread out and came toward me and my casualty. It turned out to be the battalion commander and his staff. And his name, coincidentally, was Davis, Ray Davis. Of course, he got the Medal of Honor at the Chosin Reservoir. He was my battalion commander. We brought the casualty over to the dike, and Davis just chewed my ass because I had not taken care of the patient and moved on with my platoon. And he was correct. The theory is that you take care of your patient and move on because the collecting and clearing company will come and get him. Well, they had had three hours to have done that and didn't. So I stayed with the guy and I think he survived because I was there.

We ended up at the Han River, which flows through Seoul. There were boats to take us across, but there was a village on the opposite bank and machine gun emplacements firing at us. I happened to be next to the naval gunfire officer who was calling one of the battleships out in Inchon Harbor for fire support. He gave them range changes and then told them to fire for effect. And they fired a broadside. He told me later that they fired all the 16-inch guns at one time at this village. Well, you could look up and, I'm not kidding, you could see it flying through the air and hear it because the shells were on their downward trajectory at that point. That broadside hit the village and when the smoke cleared, there was a lake full of straw and no village. It was absolutely gone.

We all got into the boats and went across. Our regiment turned north of Seoul. Our function was to catch any North Koreans who were trying to go north. The 1st and the 5th Marines were pushing them out of Seoul. We had a number of fire fights in that engagement. It was a fierce battle.

Lt. Robert J. Fleischaker, MC, 3rd Battalion, 1st Marines

We moved inland riding LVTs (Landing Vehicle Tracked), the amphibious tractors. Initially, I think the North Koreans were taken by surprise. We actually outnumbered them considerably. They brought some troops and tanks down from Seoul and there were some vicious fights that went on. There were quite a few people who were wounded in the course of the next week. The enemy had a lot of mortars, and many of the wounded we treated had been injured by mortar fragments. There were also a lot of gunshot wounds.

The resistance stiffened considerably as we approached Seoul. When we actually went through the city, the street fighting was very vicious. We had something like seventy casualties on the 25th when our troops were advancing along the main boulevard and adjacent streets through the city.

Lt. Cmdr. Chester Lessenden, MC, Regimental Surgeon, 5th Marines

The day after the landing we moved toward Kimpo Airfield. The medical companies were ashore with all their surgeons and operating theaters so the pressure was off for our definitive care of the wounded. We had a place to send our casualties. And we had a visitor—General MacArthur. He gave our colonel a Silver Star, without even knowing his name—addressed him as "that man." He picked his way among the foxholes and debris and vanished from sight. He certainly never looked at me nor at any of the wounded we were holding.

That night we were at Kimpo. Our dentist was the highest ranking—and the oldest man—in our regiment, Cmdr. Jack Kelly. He spent the night in a water-filled basement and, come daylight, he could hardly move because of his lumbago. I suggested to the division surgeon that perhaps Jack was a little old for this at forty years. So there at Kimpo, he was replaced by Morton Israel Silver, a j.g. dentist, fresh out of the City College of New York.

Mort had never done anything more active than play a little stickball in the streets of Brooklyn. He couldn't build a fire, open a can, or keep himself warm. But he was smart and eager, if not exactly gung-ho. Mort had even more to learn than I did about life with the Marines and life in the field. We became fast friends and it was my privilege to write him up for a Navy Cross later on.

We had one night to plan the Han River crossing and the advance on Seoul. I was concerned as to how we could ferry casualties [back] across this wide and deep river. Mort went with me to discuss our problem with Lt. Col. Murray. The colonel had his headquarters in the basement of a blown-out building. It was pitch-black outside, and the headquarters area was absolutely dark. Any light would draw a shot—probably from a Marine. We stepped through this light-lock where the gasoline lanterns were on. People were coming and going and the radio operators were talking. It seemed like Broadway.

Col. Murray was ordinarily a settled, calm guy, but this night he was hyper, moving and talking fast. We waited our turn, and then he listened to us for a couple of minutes. Then he suggested that we use the assault ducks [DUKWs][2] that were to haul the assault troops across to bring the casualties back on their return trip. I could then arrange for ambulances to pick up the wounded on the west side of the river and carry them on to the medical company. I would remain on the west side to receive the wounded, until the H & S [headquarters and service] company of the regiment was ferried over. The battalions would continue to use our aid station as a collecting point. It only remained for this to be explained to the battalion surgeons, provided that I could find them in the dark. But first, a word about ducks. These were like 2 ½-ton trucks, but the body was like a steel boat. They were fitted with flotation tanks that projected into the boat at odd angles. This made the loading of stretchers a tricky maneuver. We had experimented so that we knew how to do it, to accommodate the most casualties.

Mort and I went down to the river in a jeep with a driver and no headlights. We found the duck park, talked to their CO, found the battalion surgeons, explained the plan, and finished just as the artillery started. Our driver, whoever he was, must have had eyes like a cat because he delivered us safely back to our aid station. I never knew where we had been.

The next day the chain of evacuation worked well. We continued to use the ducks to ferry casualties across the river. Once across, the division turned northwest and moved up the east bank of the Han to the outskirts of Seoul. The going got rougher. The advance slowed down and more casualties began arriving. Our headquarters received some hostile fire, and one of the staff officers got some shrapnel in his derriere. We had established a rule that anyone who gave a friend anything to eat or drink after he was wounded had to stick around and clean up the vomitus. Morphine does that to people. Lo and behold! This high-ranking casualty had received a shot of brandy from a high-ranking friend. So we had a Marine Corps colonel swabbing our deck.

The next day we entered Seoul. I think the 5th and 1st Regiments went through the city abreast. The 1st put a 90mm round into every building. The 5th, probably with less opposition, took most of our part by storm. For some reason I was out after dark during this time with a driver named Dougherty, and we got lost. An eerie feeling thinking you might run into the enemy lines. We crossed a wide street and found the buildings still standing on the other side, so we knew where we were.

The 5th Regiment was headquartered at Ewah University, a Methodist Missionary school with elaborate stone buildings. The place was a mess because the North Koreans had also used it. Windows and doors were broken, floors and walls damaged, and the whole place smeared with human excrement. I think the enemy had used some of the rooms as latrines and walked in it—or may have smeared it on purpose. It's hard to know what these enemy soldiers had in mind. Our people cleaned it up with gallons of water, soap, and disinfectant so that the buildings were usable. I felt really secure behind these thick rock walls.

Lt. Col. Ray Murray, USMC, Commanding Officer, 5th Marines
I vaguely remember discussing with Dr. Lessenden how to get the casualties back from the other side of the Han [River]. Actually, the reason I was hyper was because our intelligence indicated that there was nothing on the other side of the river, opposite from where we were going to cross. There was a little hill on the other side but supposedly it was unoccupied. So I planned to make an administrative crossing rather than a standard assault crossing. In an administrative crossing, you get across as fast as you can without opposition. You don't have to form waves of assault troops and keep a distance between the waves so you don't get everybody killed at once. In an assault landing, you're prepared to fight your way across.

I sent the reconnaissance company, which was attached to me at the time, ahead over the river. They had swum across earlier in the evening just after dark. They were to scout the area and make sure there was no opposition. If there wasn't, they were to signal us to come on over. We were going to form in a column and get people across as fast as we could.

When the [reconnaissance company] got over, they didn't find anything so they signaled us to come on across. But about that time the whole hillside opened up. A battalion of North Koreans had pretty well concealed themselves in that hill.

We had to change our plans overnight and crossed the next morning. By then the opposition had left. I don't recall that we lost anybody crossing the river, which we did without difficulty. As a result, the problem of moving [casualties] back across the river never arose. We then moved up toward Seoul. It took us three or four days to take the city.

Outside of Seoul, I set up my headquarters in an abandoned building. About two o'clock in the morning, when I was fast asleep, an armor-piercing shell hit the window casement right above my head and exploded. Fortunately, it wasn't high explosive. I awoke sitting straight up with the room briefly full of flame. I discovered that I was unhurt but for a piece of shrapnel that had just hit the very tip of my nose. It was bleeding a little bit.

I didn't notice it but Les [Lessenden] saw it and said, "Would you like me to put you in for a Purple Heart?"

I said, "No, I've already got a Purple Heart and don't need another one."

That shell wounded a lot of people. It wounded my exec who was asleep on the floor. A piece of shrapnel hit him in the leg and severed a nerve. He had to be evacuated and sent home. The armor piercing part of the shell hit another man and tore most of his face off, blinding him. He survived. They rebuilt his jaw, but he was blind forever.

Hospital Corpsman Russell O'Day, Company C, 1st Engineer Battalion, 1st Marines

After we went across the Han River and went into Seoul; that's when we got the plasma. It was in a box with two bottles in it. I guess the units were about five inches long, two and a half inches in diameter. One had the powder, the other the liquid. You mixed them together and they made plasma. This box was very inconvenient to carry. So I took my two cans out of there and took some tape and taped them to the bottom of the pack on my back. I thought that was a good thing to do. And that was a mistake.

I then made the second mistake. The Marine dungarees of that time had PFC, sergeant, or corporal's stripes with big stencils on both arms. Being a hospital corpsman, all I had was HN [hospitalman rank] stenciled on my left arm. Therefore, I didn't have anything on my right arm.

The third mistake was walking in the middle of the unit single file on the outskirts of Seoul. I had a .45 as a weapon and all the Marines had carbines or M1s. If you're a sniper up in a building and you're going to shoot somebody, here's a guy with a .45. That indicates he's probably an officer. He has no rank stenciled on his arm. That indicates he's an officer. He's got these two cans on his pack. Nobody else has these two cans. And the guy is walking in the middle of the group. So a sniper took a shot and guess who he shot at? He put a bullet dead-center through the cans of plasma. He probably thought they were demolitions and if they blew, they'd get the whole lot of us. That's the only shot he got off but I learned a whole bunch of things right there.

If he had aimed at my head, he would have gotten me. He was a good shot. I got rid of that .45 and got a carbine. I stenciled some rates [rank insignia] on my right arm. I got rid of those two cans on my back and just blended in with the troops.

We went into downtown Seoul, down the main drag pulling up land mines in front of the tanks. I was over by a building trying to keep out of the way when a guy got hit out in the middle of the street. He must have had his rifle up at port arms or something because it hit his M1 first, shattering it. The bullet, or whatever it was, went on and hit him in the chest. I went out there and dragged him from the middle of the road and up into a building. He was a typical Marine. At that time, they taught Marines in boot camp that if you lost your weapon, they'd take $67 dollars out of your pay. And they drummed that into Marines' heads. Well, this guy's weapon is shattered out there in the middle of the road, and I have him up in that building where I'm patching him up. All the time he kept moaning and groaning, "Get my weapon. I lost my weapon. Go get my weapon." I knew I wasn't going out in the street to get that rifle.

Gunnery Sgt. Garrison O. Gigg, Company C, 1st Engineer Battalion, 1st Marines
Back in those days they had what they called the engineer tank infantry assault. The engineers would go out and we'd clear the road of mines. We'd check the bridges before the tanks went over. After we gave the OK, the tanks would come up and start peppering away and moving on down the road. In a lot of cases we used to ride in the bow gunner's seat in the tank looking through the viewing ports for any depressions or mounds in the road that might indicate a mine. We'd then pop out of the hatch, probe that area, and then crawl back into the hatch and keep on moving. The infantry would then come up right after the tanks. They called this the engineer tank infantry assault.

Seoul was a house-by-house type of urban warfare. It was just like clearing a town no worse or no better than the Army was doing during World War II going through France after D-Day. You'd run into a village and then have to clear it house by house. And that's what Seoul was except that the North Koreans had barricaded the streets with rice bags and had antitank guns and machine guns set up behind these barricades. What we did was to clear the house up to the barricade. Then we'd have to clear the barricade and then continue down the road.

We were working on our second or third barricade this day, and I don't really know what happened. I just know that a shell exploded and the next thing I know I'm lying there and can't see with blood all over the place.

I thought, "Well, I'm dead."

Somebody hollered, "Corpsman!" and he was right there in a matter of seconds dragging me off the street.

When I was hit I left my M1 laying out in the middle of the street. As the corpsman dragged me in I kept hollering, "God dammit, I gotta go out there and get my rifle. Go back out and get my rifle, doc."

He said, "You sonofabitch, I hauled your ass in here; I'm not going back out for your damn rifle!"

The next thing I knew I woke up in a battalion aid station. It wasn't until forty-six years later when I met him again that Russell O'Day, the corpsman, told me exactly what happened. All I know is that I owe him what life I have.

Lt.(j.g.) Henry Litvin, MC, 2nd Battalion, 5th Marines
The day after the landing I found myself in a clearing near some farmhouses. There I met Col. Roise and other officers and men. It was our second day in combat

when I became aware of something called Headquarters and Service Company. That day I met Dr. Chester Klein and the corpsmen I'd be working with. He had been in combat at the Naktong River. I got the feeling afterward that when Korea broke out, they shoved a lot of doctors over there with no training or indoctrination. At the time I felt scared half out of my mind. Afterward I learned that this was not an unusual experience for doctors.

The first night we stayed in a little hut in the town of Inchon. The second night we slept in an open field. About two or three in the morning, everybody awoke to a very strange sound. It was the sound of tanks. It was a sound I'll never forget. Everybody got ready to do something. There was a lot of gunfire and then there were three loud explosions. The next day when we filed by the three tanks, we were told that Marines with "bazookas" had taken them out. They were still smoking and there were the burned bodies of North Koreans.

Something really important happened between Inchon and Seoul. Our battalion took Kimpo Airfield. The battalion headquarters company, which I was part of, was not in the lead. The rifle companies were in the lead and we came along behind them. But you felt like you were walking onto this airfield and you knew the enemy was around because you heard rifle fire and bullets whizzing. But it was getting dark. We were told to put our aid station there and we did. There didn't seem to be a whole lot going on. I guess we should have dug in but instead we got some litters and just flopped down on them.

In the middle of the night our eyes opened up. If you can imagine being flat on your back and looking up and seeing all these tracers crisscrossing the sky. That was quite an experience. And there was another sound you can't imagine, the sound of a battleship's 16-inch shells flying overhead. They sounded like freight trains. I was scared to death. Someone said, "Don't worry, Doc. They're going overhead." A day or two later, when we moved, we came across these huge craters and I was told they were the results of the 16-inch shells.

The first night we were in what looked like a bombed-out store near the English legation in Inchon. They brought wounded in and we treated them. The second night we were out in the field. The third and fourth nights we were still around Inchon in the open. Between Kimpo and Seoul was a series of fields. I was told, "Doc, there's your aid station." So that's where we worked. It was warm so I don't remember tents being set up. We were out in the open most of the time.

One thing that's bothered the hell out of me these past fifty years is that I don't even remember plasma or IV fluid, though I'm sure we used IV fluids. I just can't bring back a visual picture. There had to have been plasma and IV saline, but it's blocked out of my memory. I can remember wounds. I can remember battle dressings. I can remember sulfa.

I was literally grasping at straws to treat shock. Stop bleeding, keep them flat, and evacuate them to the rear fast. I never knew about MASH until years later when the show came out. I remember sitting with my wife watching it and being furious. They were laughing and I never remember much laughter. I don't remember any laughter where we were.

As for the concept of medical evacuation, I had a basic assumption. There has to be a rear; I know I'm close to the front so there's gotta be somebody behind. Looking back, the wounded were evacuated by jeep and ambulance very fast. Patients didn't stay at the aid station long. To this day, I've never talked to a senior medical officer who could tell me what the evacuation route was. I'm only guessing that the casualties went back to regiment, then back to division or back to a medical company.

My medical unit consisted of two hospital chiefs and maybe eight to ten corpsmen of various grades at battalion level. Each of the three rifle companies had several corpsmen. What worried us was getting a call from a company saying, "Doc, we're out of corpsmen." And then we'd have to look around and send someone up to the rifle companies, which was like a death sentence. As it turned out, when all this was over, I thought back on things. I had over a 100 percent replacement of corpsmen. The corpsmen up with the rifle companies were getting shot at an alarming rate, and we were sending up replacements all the time. Had I had some training, I might have known the proper military procedure for picking replacements. But it seemed that the corpsmen I'd run into at the battalion aid level kind of stayed put and it was only in a desperate situation where I had to send one of them up. I didn't do much of the sending between Inchon and Seoul. It was only afterward when Dr. Klein left and a new doctor named Sparks joined us that I had to do the sending.

I recall being under a blanket with the chief corpsman and a flashlight. He was writing the names of these two blond kids who were just off the ship. I remember talking with them and telling them they were going up to Dog, Easy, or Fox Company. And off they went. The next morning I got word from the CO.

"We need more corpsmen."

"I just sent you two."

"They're dead."

I took two kids and sent them up to die. I always felt personally responsible. There's a lot of guilt associated with that.

Moving toward Seoul after Kimpo was the worst fighting in terms of numbers of casualties. They were coming in at a terrible rate. We were working day and night, day and night. I remember jeeps with one or two litters on them and box ambulances. There was always a steady stream coming in. We were literally stopping bleeding, splinting fractures, giving something for pain, and sending them back. It seemed at battalion level you were just doing first aid. I don't know that I had any suture material and, even had there been any, you were never clean enough to do anything. It was an unbelievably chaotic nightmare. Again, at the time, I simply reacted to what was in front of me.

There were a number of times when guys died in your arms or if not your arms, you were kneeling next to them. Many times, the last word out of their mouth was Mom. Not God, not country but Mom. Memories like that stay in your mind and never go away.

Notes
[1]A smokeless, slow-burning powder used as a propellant in munitions.
[2]The amphibious truck developed during World War II carried the manufacturer's code DUKW. [D (1942); U (utility truck amphibious; K (all-wheel-drive); W (dual rear axles)].

3

Chosin

*B*y *late September 1950, Gen. Douglas MacArthur's brilliantly planned and executed landing at Inchon and the swift recapture of Seoul had dramatically changed the complexion of the war. United Nations troops, once faced with annihilation by the North Koreans, were on the offensive in South Korea chasing the fleeing enemy back across the 38th Parallel. It was then that President Truman, supported by a UN resolution to establish a free and united Korea, made the fateful decision not only to punish the aggressors who had started the war but to liberate the communist North, thereby insuring the reunification of the two Koreas.*

The coup de grâce was to be another landing, this time on North Korea's east coast. Extreme tides had bedeviled the Inchon planners. At Wonsan, the problem was a heavily mined harbor that delayed the landing for nearly two weeks. As the mine-clearing proceeded, the Marines aimlessly cruised up and down the Korean coast aboard LSTs and other vessels in what the men derisively called "Operation Yo Yo."

When the Marines finally disembarked at Wonsan, the port had already been captured by ROK (Republic of Korea) and UN troops. Greeting them was a sign reading "Bob Hope welcomes you." What these troops could not know was that within a few short weeks the war in Korea would again change dramatically. As the Marines were working their way north, they were moving ever closer to the Manchurian border. Gone was their traditional role of conducting operations from and near the sea. They now encountered rugged mountain terrain, a brutal winter climate, and finally thousands of quilt-uniformed Chinese who suddenly descended upon them in hordes. Today, places and events are frozen in the memories of the campaign's survivors—Sudong, Chosin Reservoir, Yudam-ni, East Hill, Toktong Pass, Hagaru-ri, Koto-ri.

* * *

First Encounter

Hospital corpsman Bill Davis, stiff from being cooped up aboard an LST for nearly two weeks as Wonsan Harbor was being cleared, looked forward to taking on the foe in another glorious amphibious operation. Although the landing turned out to be bloodless and anticlimactic, his 7th Marines would be the first Americans to encounter a new and far more numerous enemy.

When we got to Wonsan we were all hyped up for the landing but, in the interim, the South Koreans had crossed the 38th Parallel and occupied the place. When we landed, there was a great big sign that said, "Bob Hope and the 1st Marine Air Wing Welcome the 1st Marine Division to Wonsan."

Col. [Homer] Litzenberg, the regimental commander, was mad, to say the least. He had had this vision of charging ashore. Marines don't want to come ashore and find Bob Hope there.

Litzenberg said, "We're getting out of here." So we marched to Hamhung without stopping, maybe thirty-five miles from where we landed.

When we got to Hamhung, they put us in some kind of warehouse, and we just sat around and waited for something to happen. The popular song of the Korean War was "Goodnight Irene," and we sang it in this big warehouse for hours.

A guy named Kelly had been an engineer on a railroad in Chicago. When we found a railroad train outside, someone thought it would be nice to be able to drive it. Kelly said that if we could get some wood he could. So we went out, found wood, and old Kelly got it started. We all had a ride up the track, not going anywhere in particular, just back and forth. This went on until they came and dragged us off. But it killed the time.

We weren't there two days and then we began to form up for what would be the move north. It was fairly calm until we got to a place called Sudong. This was early November, and it was the first time, it turns out, the Chinese were actually in combat with the 1st Marine Division. The 1st Battalion, 7th Marines, was the first unit to fight with them, and it was at night when they attacked us. They had us surrounded with bugles, loudspeakers, and green flares. That was a tough night and one hell of a battle. We worked all night long because we had one hell of a lot of casualties. We'd had firefights and casualties before but never anything like this.

One of our wounded was a guy named Archie van Winkle, a platoon sergeant of the 3rd platoon. He had been shot in the belly and was lying on the deck when I got to him. He was very badly hit, and I had to bandage him in four different places. All I got was a thready pulse. I didn't think he was going to make it down off that hill, and I wrote on his little toe tag that he was KIA. Well, obviously he wasn't because he got down off the hill, recovered, stayed in the Marines, and eventually became a colonel. Later he was awarded the Medal of Honor for what he did on that hill.

All we had were bandages and morphine. We had to get the casualties back to the battalion aid station before they could get IVs and what have you. Our company, which might have had one hundred fifty men, maybe a little more than that with the mortar and machine gun people, took thirty or forty casualties that night. That's a hell of a lot of casualties for one battle. The

Chinese then disappeared, and we never saw them again until we got up to the Chosin Reservoir.

I recall an incident that took place right after Sudong. Some Koreans had outside brick ovens. They cooked on them and also hid in them, whether from the North Koreans or us. A civilian told our translator that there was somebody inside one of those ovens who had been hurt. They sent me. It was a girl about twelve years old who was wounded in the hand and had gangrene up to her elbow. I knew damn well that it had advanced far enough so that it would take her arm at least or kill her at worst. But I put sulfa powder and a bandage on anyway. I left some bandages with the civilians and we took off. Afterward, those people had nothing, absolutely nothing. That was one of the sad parts of being a corpsman over there.

* * *

Cold Weather Combat

Late fall and winter of 1950 in North Korea was the coldest on record, arctic in its intensity. The mercury plummeted almost overnight, with temperatures dropping to nearly thirty-five degrees below zero. Merely sustaining life in such weather was arduous enough. Keeping warm, eating, drinking, and even relieving oneself—all normal functions in a temperate climate—became anything but routine. For Marines fighting off swarms of Chinese bent on exterminating them, most everything began to appear hopeless.

As oil and grease thickened and then froze, rifles, carbines, and machine guns ceased to function. Mortar base plates became brittle and cracked. Artillery recoil mechanisms balked, drastically reducing the rate of fire. Unless jeep and truck engines were kept running, crankcase oil took on the viscosity of molasses. Batteries died, canned rations solidified, and canteen water froze. Dehydration is a given in a sun-baked desert, but no one could have anticipated dehydration in the cold. Unable to drink, men sucked snow to relieve their thirst, further lowering body temperature and making them more susceptible to hypothermia. And the greatest by-product of the cold—frostbite—downed more men than Chinese bullets.

Gunnery Sgt. Garrison Gigg, attached to the 1st Engineer Battalion of the 1st Marines, recalls the torment of cold weather combat.

Weapons

We learned real quickly that you couldn't use Lubriplate (white grease) or oil on rifles and machine guns, absolutely none, because both would instantly freeze. Then you had to take your Ka-Bar [knife] or bayonet and try to scrape it off the bolt to get it to function. The bolt and everything had to be dry.

The artillery also had a heck of a problem. Normally, the guns would fire, then recoil and go back into battery, ready for another shell in a matter of a second. A good crew could get off fifteen, twenty, or twenty-five rounds a minute. But the cold weather was so bad on the artillery that when they fired, it sometimes took five minutes or longer for the gun to come back into battery so the crew could load another round. As a result, we lost 65 to 70 percent of our firepower.

Clothing

If you were going to start from scratch and go from the skin out, you had your Marine Corps issue skivvies—[boxer] shorts and T-shirt. Some guys had long underwear—long johns— some didn't. The majority of us that came in at Wonsan didn't have the long underwear. Over a period of time we managed to scrounge up some. I remember having a pair but I don't ever remember changing my underwear for ten or twelve days from when the Chinese hit us at Chosin until we got back down aboard ship and took a shower.

If you had a winter shirt—your greens—you wore that. Then you wore heavy green trousers if you had them. If not, you wore dungaree trousers. And if you had those, you wore those besides the green trousers. Then you wore any sweatshirts or anything else on the top. They issued a pair of what they called cold weather pants with the parkas. They were windproof. You put that over the top of everything else you had on.

Then you wore the parka, which was about knee length and had buttons and a belt. If you got your own size you were lucky. If you didn't, you took what was available. It was not fleece lined but had a carpeting kind of material. They called it a fur lining but it was more nappy than fluffy. You can get some jackets like that today from L.L. Bean.

Then you wore your helmet and gloves with wool liners on the inside. Those were separate. You put on the wool liners and then the outer glove, which was made of a kind of canvas and leather. The top part was like a boat canvas, and the palms were like a work glove an electrician or a lumberjack might wear. It was not real heavy leather but a supple leather. Both hands had the trigger finger built into it as part of the glove. The top part was cloth and the palm of the glove was leather. With the glove on, it was extremely difficult to get the trigger finger through the trigger guard so a lot of the guys would cut that part of the glove off. Sometimes that caused the trigger finger to freeze to the trigger. It was like sticking your tongue on a light pole in the winter.

Headgear

We had caps with a little bill and ear flaps you could tie down under your chin. It was fleece lined and Marine Corps green. Over that you wore your helmet or your parka and your helmet on top of that. The problem with wearing the hat and even the parka was that if you were in a fire fight, running a ridge, or whatever you were doing, you needed to be able to correspond with whoever was next to you. But, in some cases, it was snowing so hard you couldn't see. So you had to go by voice command. You also needed to hear the snow crunch if someone was trying to sneak up on you. We'd put out concertina wire with cans on it and if someone tried to come through the wire, they'd make noise. But with that hat on, with the ear muffs tied down, and the parka tied down over your ears, it was difficult to hear, so you had to undo those. And when you did, it exposed your ears to frostbite. A lot of the frostbite cases are having problems now. I'm having problems with both of my ears from frostbite. My ears are starting to point like a Martian's. They're not black, but they are exceedingly brown.

Footgear

We wore the so-called shoepacs. They were all rubber and black. You've seen Mickey Mouse wearing his boots? That's about what they looked like. In fact, they called them Mickey Mouse boots. They were uninsulated rubber, as I recall, with a removable felt inner sole. You had two pairs of those. You kept one pair next to your body trying to keep them dry or to dry them out after they got wet. And the other pair you kept in your boots. The whole idea for these boots was to keep your feet warm. As long as you were walking it was great. They worked perfectly well. As a matter of fact, they worked so well that your feet would perspire and actually made water. The felt pads then soaked up that perspiration. Then, when you stopped, the water in the shoepacs froze. You usually wore two pairs of socks, sometimes three, whatever you had. They'd get wet and freeze to your skin. When you took your boots off, you'd take the skin off with it.

Frostbite

I didn't realize I had a problem until I got back down to the Bean Patch [Masan] and my feet started to hurt and the skin started to peel and crack. But my frostbite was not as bad as some. The problems really started about fifteen years ago, and now it's getting progressively worse. Some days are worse than others. When the circulation stops you also lose sensation in your feet. But when you start walking or rubbing your feet, the tingling begins when the circulation begins to come back.

Some of the symptoms are drying skin, rotting, cracking largely due to lack of circulation. I've lost three toenails on one foot and half a big toe. I've also lost the big toenail on the other foot. My feet are always cracked and blistering. Apparently the frostbite does something to the capillaries and smaller vessels in your feet the older you get. As time wears on, they get worse and worse until you have no circulation, and eventually they drop off. It's almost like getting gangrene. We have a fellow who heads our "Chosin Few" cold injury committee who now walks around in specially made shoes. His feet are probably five inches long. The rest of his feet have just rotted away. They've had to cut away parts of his feet and he's had multiple surgeries over the years.

The infantry guys in the line companies who were running the ridges were constantly on the move with the sweat and the cold. We had a couple of Marines in the foxhole next to us. A corpsman hollered for litter bearers. I crawled out of my hole and, with a couple of other guys, went over and lugged these men out. Their feet were black. They had been out there sweeping the ridges while we were farther on down the mountain protecting the convoy—the line of march—and the MSR, the main supply route.

Food and personal hygiene

We had a heck of a hard time eating. Our C-rations were frozen and the only way you could possibly get them warm was if you were lucky enough to have a bulldozer, a truck, or a jeep nearby. You put the C-ration can on the engine block so it would thaw. And then when you opened the can, it might be partially thawed or it might not be. You then scraped away what was thawed and ate that. Then you would thaw it out some more and eat that, so you were constantly eating frozen food that was probably frozen and rethawed God knows how many times before you got through the can.

We had no purification systems with us so the only water we drank was melted snow, or we simply ate snow which was probably full of *e-coli,* botulism, salmonella, or whatever. A lot of guys, including me, had a very bad case of what I called stomach-rot. Imagine you've got diarrhea and you've got all these clothes on. You're in a foxhole and the head is some boulders some four or five meters behind your foxhole.

One night we were in an area with some downed trees so we had some cover. You knew that as soon as you picked your head out of the foxhole the Chinese were going to shoot at you. So you unbuttoned all your clothes and got ready to go down to the head. Then you made a dash for it. When you got there, you dropped your drawers, did your business, and reached for your C-ration toilet paper. By the time you got the toilet paper, you had nothing but frozen dingle berries. You pulled up your pants and went back up to the foxhole. In about fifteen minutes, your body heat would melt the feces you had left. You came out of there with ulcers on your rear end and you smelled something terrible. But, of course, it was so damned cold, you couldn't smell anything anyhow. A lot of people walked down that mountain range with ulcerated rear ends from the cold. And that's not fiction; it's fact.

I don't remember shaving from the time we left Wonsan and started up to Sudong where we ran into our first Chinese. I cannot remember having any way of shaving or cleaning myself or doing anything from the time we first got hit until we got aboard ship again. I don't even remember that first shower, and don't know what happened to my clothes.

Burying the Dead

We had a lot of dead at Yudam-ni, Hagaru [ri], and at Koto-ri. We were getting near the tail end and were attacking toward the sea. The vehicles were loaded with wounded and there was not room for all the dead. And the Marine Corps always says you take your wounded and your dead with you. At Hagaru [ri] and Koto-ri that was impossible. The worst thing was witnessing the digging of a mass grave there at Hagaru [ri]. We used explosives to try to soften up the ground, but we just couldn't do it. It was so damned hard. We welded teeth on the dozer blades and, in combination with explosives, we tried to soften up the ground. There were some huts in that area where there had been fires and the ground was soft underneath. We bulldozed the huts down and eventually got the graves dug. We buried two hundred Marines and Royal Marines in that grave.

At Koto-ri we dug a light airstrip so C-47s could come in. The first day we had that strip operational, 700 wounded were evacuated. At Koto-ri we dug another grave and left 125 more bodies there. That's the stuff that haunts you and you can never get rid of it.

* * *

Frozen in Memory

Lt.(j.g.) Henry Litvin, MC, now a "veteran" of Inchon, Kimpo Airport, and Seoul, recalls how he cared for the sick and wounded of the 2nd Battalion, 5th Marines, and survived an unmerciful environment where it always seemed that the very next moment would be his last.

From mid-October to early November, we slowly worked our way up east of the [Chosin] Reservoir. Patrols that went out brought in Chinese prisoners every once in a while. And then suddenly the weather turned cold. I was having breakfast one morning, gulping down some eggs. When I went to get the coffee, it was frozen. I couldn't imagine coffee freezing. We didn't have a thermometer but it had to have been well below zero. It occurred to me right then that practicing medicine was going to be a difficult thing.

I attended a meeting of Marine officers somewhere up on the way to Hagaru-ri, where they talked about the move we were going to make north. Many things were discussed but the thing that stuck in my mind was a high-ranking Marine officer's comments about frostbite. I vividly remember him talking about it the same way he'd view a sunburn, namely, something that could be avoided. So when I first heard about frostbite, I figured these guys were going to get into trouble. But frostbite couldn't be avoided when you were pinned down, had sweaty feet, and couldn't change your socks. If you were wounded and lying there, you couldn't change your socks. If you were wounded and strapped to a vehicle, your sweat froze.

In hindsight, it's a miracle that anybody avoided frostbite. It didn't resemble trench foot as in World War I, when feet were cold and wet for long periods of time. We were wearing shoepacs which were rubberized boots. If you walked twenty feet in them, your feet started to perspire. And if you stopped, they'd freeze. I was in a position where I could maybe change my socks once a day. But there were a lot of troops who could not change their socks when they were pinned down or fighting. Changing your socks at twenty below with a stiff breeze is murder, but they did it. We'd go up and down the line telling people to stamp their feet, change their socks, and keep moving.

As for clothing, everybody had long johns, two layers of trousers, those flannel shirts, maybe a field jacket. Everybody had a parka and gloves. When we tried to deal with the wounded, we'd take our gloves off and our fingers would freeze.

Water was also a problem in that intense cold. Everybody was dehydrated. I had never experienced such an overwhelming thirst. You read about the exhaustion and the cold, but you never read about the dehydration. There was nowhere to get a drink. Up in those mountains the humidity is low. We were losing a lot of moisture from our skin. Once I grabbed a canteen and found myself trying to suck ice; the contents were frozen solid. There were water trucks down south, but I never saw them up north. We had to melt snow to make coffee. For days we went without any food. We were starved but not hungry. At one point someone found a cache of Tootsie Rolls so we loaded up on Tootsie Rolls.

Everybody had runny noses. It ran into their moustaches and froze. Everybody was filthy, grimy, dirty, and crawling with lice. And can you imagine having to move your bowels. The wind's blowing twenty or thirty miles an hour and it's forty below zero and you have to go. You do what you have to do and you don't have time to wipe. Peeing was easy.

If you were treating a wound, you'd cut through the clothing to where the wound was, or you'd put a battle dressing over the clothes and make sure the wound wasn't leaking blood. I remember vividly one Marine after Yudam-ni. When he approached the tent, it looked like he had a block of pink cotton candy sitting on his shoulder. I couldn't imagine what I was looking at. As he got closer, I noticed it was pink, frothy ice. I broke it off and then realized he had been hit and had a bleeder above his ear. Frozen blood is frothy pink. It was actively bleeding and freezing, bleeding and freezing.

It seemed that the intense cold inhibited bleeding. The wounds we saw had already been wrapped by corpsmen in the companies. If the battle dressing was in place, even over their clothing, and there was no leaking blood, we just checked the battle dressing and left the wounds alone.

I saw head wounds and leg wounds. There were some belly wounds. There were countless extremity wounds that blur in my mind. There was one guy with a sucking chest wound, and I remember getting an idea. I said, "Does anybody have a rubber?" Then thinking, "Who would have condoms up here?" One guy had one. I unrolled it, taped it over the wound, and cut some little slits in it thinking that if he developed a pressure pneumothorax, the air would get out. I was able to get this kid out on a helicopter.

Remember, the helicopters then were not like the ones in Vietnam. There was a bubble for the pilot and, if there was a guy on a litter, half of him stuck out. He was the only one I got out by helicopter. We saw helicopters that looked like the wind had dashed them against the sides of the mountains. They looked like broken little toys. There weren't a lot of helicopters flying.

The Chinese attacked at night or when it snowed, for the most part, often announcing their presence with whistles and bugles. But the thing I remember most were the mortar explosions. All night long you heard them. And all those explosions didn't do much to improve my hearing. I had tinnitus then, which I didn't pay much attention to, but I'm sure my deafness today is related to that. After seeing all the bullet holes in the tent canvas, you wanted to go outside and stretch and look around. In the morning, I remember seeing hundreds of unexploded Chinese mortar shells on the ground.

We worked at night because that's when most of the wounded were coming in. We had no table. Most of the time we were on our knees or bent over somebody on the ground or on a litter doing some procedure.

I never saw a pair of sterile gloves in Korea. I never saw forceps or anything sterile in Korea. The only things sterile were the battle dressings and the morphine syrettes.

We never knew how long it was going to be until the wounded person could get to further care. So we protected them by using sulfa. I think it was more for ourselves. We were doing something. At the time you didn't think too much about it. You just did it. We never had IV fluids at any time at our battalion level. They would have frozen solid.

Down south when you treated the wounded, you checked for bleeding, splinted them, gave them something for pain, and evacuated them. Up north you did the same things, but you had to hold onto your patients because there was no way to get them out and the numbers kept growing. Soon we were getting hundreds of casualties yet there was no place to put them. When we had wounded and no place to send them, we'd push them to the side or get them into another tent if there was one—and usually there wasn't—or out in the open covered with a tarp. Or we'd put them in a truck and stack them like cordwood. We stacked them the way the dead were stacked. We tied them on the hoods of jeeps or trucks. There was no regiment to send them back to. We were the end of the line—the rear guard. If men could walk, they walked.

I remember a lieutenant. He looked like a very young kid—blond hair. They brought him in and put him down. There was a bullet hole in the side of his helmet. He was lying on the snow and breathing but not conscious. I removed his helmet and his brains spilled out like oatmeal onto the snow. He was still breathing and had a pulse. The bullet had entered and ricocheted around the inside of his helmet. I remember putting the helmet back and saying, "Move him out there." These are memories that stay in your head forever.

We went days and nights without rest. We were exhausted. There were few times when you could get horizontal because it was at night when the casualties were coming. During the day you were moving so you went days with no real sleep. When we stacked the wounded on trucks, you thought, "Thank God, at least they are getting to lie down." But I'm sure many wounded froze. The fact that I kept walking, like most of the guys at the aid station, helped me avoid freezing. If you stopped and sat, you'd freeze. I can't prove that many of the wounded froze, but I suspect that's what must have happened.

I don't know what we would have done without the corpsmen. There were corpsmen who had been seasoned in World War II and there were corpsmen as green as I was. They didn't have to fight with rifles but went where they were called. They were always on the go. I wasn't up with the companies to see them, but at the rate they were getting hit, these guys were unsung heroes. When the call went out for corpsmen, they went.

One memory stands out. It was November 27th, about 10 P.M,. Our unit was point battalion for the Division and we were a few miles northwest of Yudam-ni. There had been some firing during the day and we had stopped for the night. Seven or eight of us were sitting around in a tent. There was a lantern going. It was cold and the wind was blowing. Suddenly this guy slides down the hill right through the side of our tent with no shoepacs on, no helmet. He says, "Where's the colonel? Where's the colonel? I need to tell him. They've overrun us! Fox Company has been overrun." It seems the Chinese were atop the hill just above us.

With that, all of us flew out of the tent, door or no door, right through the sides. I rolled down across a little road, down a gully toward a frozen little creek. It was dark but I hid behind a bunch of bushes and lay there shaking. The attack had started and there was a racket—whistles, bugles, rockets, explosions, and firing. People were shouting. "What do I do?" I thought. I couldn't see what was going on. I asked myself, "What am I supposed to do?" I lay there with another guy. I never knew who he was.

After a while we heard, "Corpsman! Corpsman!" With that, all of us moved back to the aid station and began to treat the wounded. No matter how scared I was, and believe me, I was scared, when you did your job you weren't helpless. Perhaps the sprinkling of sulfa into their wounds was more for me than it was for the patient. In a bombardment when you were doing nothing but waiting for a shell to drop, you were completely helpless and that was traumatic as hell and the most devastating thing in the world. There were days on the way back when we'd look up toward dawn and see light shining everywhere through the canvas and realize that the tent was full of bullet holes. But I understood that as long as I was doing something, I didn't sit there like a shaking lump of jelly. Work was a great thing for the doc—it overcame his terror.

On the morning of the 28th of November the decision was made to move back to Hungnam. The 2nd Battalion, 5th Marines, became the rear guard. As we began moving back to Yudam-ni, we came under fire. I remember there was nowhere to hide. Mortar rounds and fire were coming in. We had seen Chinese coming over the mountains and my feeling was, "Let's get the hell out of here. Let's keep going *that* way."

We didn't move a quarter of a mile before we saw Chinese pouring over the hill we just left. They were all around us. We felt they were going to overrun us then or in the next hour. I felt like I was literally waiting to die.

Somewhere about halfway between Yudam-ni and Hagaru [ri] was Toktong Pass, which I didn't particularly notice on the way up. I have a vivid freeze-frame of it in my mind's eye today for the following reason.

During the days and nights we were on the road between Yudam-ni and Toktong Pass, we were on a little road carved into the side of a mountain. To our left was a several-hundred-foot mountain, and to our right was a drop of hundreds and hundreds of feet. The days were short that time of year so it was dark most of the time. Most of the time during the day we were in the shadow of this mountain. I don't remember much sunlight or I wasn't aware that we were in darkness most of the time until we got to Toktong Pass.

We had been moving slowly. We'd stop and wait until the enemy had been cleared. Then we'd move and then stop. We spent days and nights on that road. When we got to Toktong Pass, looking forward I could see a turn in the road. The hill on our left kind of fell away and I watched troops ahead of me—six, eight, or ten men—get on the right side of a vehicle and at someone's signal they took off and started to run. When I finally got to that point of departure, I saw this brilliant, white, snow-covered field in brilliant sunshine. It was like being backstage in a theater where people stand before going onstage. And at a signal, we began running in the wide open across this brilliant white snow field, crouched over. It seemed quiet but for the sound of bullets flying. They make a buzz when they go by—a high-pitched "bzz, bzz," like bees. About halfway across we stopped because we found two Marines in the snow.

Quickly we ran to the back of a crackerbox ambulance. When we opened it up, we found there was absolutely no room. We had somebody on the fenders, and there was literally no place to put these two fellows.

Then there was a moment that seemed to stretch out forever when the driver was looking at me. "What do we do?"

It seemed like forever between his question and my saying, "Go!" It couldn't have been more than a split-second, but it felt like an eternity with that white, bright sun, the white snow, bullets singing, being nakedly exposed out in the open.

It seemed like there were a thousand things coming in at you. If that ambulance goes, that's your invisible shield protecting you from the bullets. You want to run but you have to stay with these guys. All of a sudden that road with the hills to the left and the drop off to the right seemed like a safer place. And then off went the ambulance. We waited for another vehicle, got the wounded aboard, and then took off and ran until we caught up with the line of troops on the road.

When I was a kid I used to love when it snowed. It meant we could go sledding and play in it. For years after I got back I felt sadness and anxiety when it began to snow, and I could never figure out why until one day it occurred to me. When it snowed up there in the north, the Corsairs wouldn't be flying and there would be no air cover. We were on our own.

For years afterwards, I kept models of [F4U] Corsairs. They're up in the attic somewhere now. Those gull-winged planes gave us close air support. It was like having a whole artillery regiment where you wanted them when you wanted them. We saw them in action in the south and thanked God for them. But up north, when we were encircled and felt isolated and helpless, to have those guys fly by at eye level and see their faces smiling, and have them give us the "thumbs up" sign, that really made us feel good. You could see them napalming, rocketing, and machine gunning the enemy. You knew they were blasting our way out. They were literally rescuing angels. I've always thought that if it hadn't been for the Corsairs, we might not have gotten out.

On the way down between Yudam-ni and Hagaru [ri], someone brought in two or three Chinese prisoners. These guys were dressed in quilted uniforms and were wearing sneakers. You never saw frostbite like this—huge bullae on their feet.[1] You can't be out there wearing sneakers like these guys wore. They just froze. Some of their wounded had been treated by their docs, who packed their wounds with gauze to get some hemostasis. We used pressure dressings on our men. We couldn't do anything for the Chinese and, when we moved out, we left their wounded behind.

For days we were moving down from Yudam-ni to Hagaru [ri] and the Marines were fighting like hell. I don't know how many days we walked. I never rode. I always walked. But I noticed that as we got closer to Hagaru [ri], everybody began changing the way they walked. When we entered Hagaru [ri], we were marching like military men.

At Hagaru [ri], all our wounded were turned over to Regiment. There was an airstrip so they were able to fly them out. When there was an air drop, you had to run to get out of the way because when those things came down—food and military supplies—they'd flatten tents and go right through huts. But it was exciting. It made you feel good. They hadn't forgotten us.

On December 6th, troops had been filing out of Hagaru [ri] all day on the way to Koto-ri. By nightfall, there were few troops left to defend our position from the same number of Chinese we had been fighting for three days. That's when they brought in Capt. Uel Peters [commanding officer, Fox Company] sitting on a litter holding a tourniquet. His leg was out like that, a compound fracture, displaced, and his flesh was glowing. We were in a tent with a Coleman lantern which didn't provide great light. "What the hell's that?" I asked. One of my corpsmen told me it was white phosphorus. I thought, "What the hell do you do with white phosphorus?"

He gave me a solution, told me it was copper sulfate, and told me to dab it on the wound. I remember dabbing it for hours until all the glow went away. That corpsman knew about white phosphorus from the South Pacific battles of World War II.

Peters had flesh and bone exposed but his wound was not actively bleeding. In fact, I don't remember seeing any active arterial bleeding while I was up there but for that guy who had the block of ice on his shoulder. Peters subsequently lost that leg. The thought has many times gone through my head, "Could I have done something different?" But I guess I did the best I could. These kinds of thoughts stay with you.

About half a city block away from our aid station, East Hill began to rise. It reminds me of that Prudential ad with the Rock of Gibraltar. There were a lot of hills but it stuck out. It was a big, ominous, dark, forbidding presence. To me, it has to be symbolic because that's where many of our troops were dying.

That same day—the 6th—everybody was funneling out of that valley blowing up supplies we didn't want to leave for the enemy. We were headed for a place called Koto-ri. Well, we were the last ones left that night. I was thinking, "We're dead!" All the troops who had been fighting off the Chinese had gone and we were still there. And we had the same enemy to deal with. That was a night! That was the night they brought in Karle Seydel. Karle Seydel was the guy who took me under his wing on the ship before Inchon and had shown me the ropes. He had taught me how to put my pack on…. He was a Marine's Marine and yet he stood on the railing of that ship going to Inchon reciting poetry. He was important to me because he reached out to me. "Don't worry, Doc. You're with amtracs and you're not with the infantry. You'll be all right."

They brought Karle in and he had a bullet in his forehead. I remember…so many dead, so many wounded. But this guy I knew better than I knew anybody else. I spent more time with him. It seemed so terrible. I wanted to do something, but his face was gray and he was dead. Every Memorial Day after that I'd reminisce, and Karle Seydel's name would come up. I'd remember him there at Hagaru [ri]. He wasn't the first dead Marine I saw, but he was a very important Marine. I have a hard time with his death to this day.

Many times I had the feeling of utter hopelessness. There's no way to get out of here. We're too far away from the sea. We're seventy miles up in the mountains and we're completely surrounded. And they could have destroyed us but didn't. Maybe the Chinese knew they were up against Marines who knew a thing or two about how to fight.

Another thing amazes me. To have walked the distance we did out of there is mind-boggling until you consider the Marines who ran up and down the hills covering us. It's one thing to make the hike but how about the guys who were running up and down tangling with the enemy on top of those ridges!

There is one view I have where we came around the bend of a road and all of a sudden I could see a plain in the distance. There were no longer peaks and valleys. It was a broad plain. We were at the bottom of a mountain range and prepared to head down toward the sea. They put us on trains—flatcars—wood-burning trains—and took us the last ten or twenty miles. It was at night. You were sitting on a flatcar with one Marine right up against you and another right behind. We were numb with exhaustion. A shower of sparks from the locomotive was falling on us, and I remember watching the sparks burning holes in my parka—pretty, orange holes burning in my parka.

We got to Hungnam and showers and food. I don't have a memory of seeing the ships until we were getting ready to board them. Being pulled aboard those ships, I remember thinking, "The Navy didn't abandon me. The Navy didn't forget about me." When I got to the top of the ladder, a couple of sailors grabbed me and I went sliding across the deck as happy as a lark. The first time I walked into a bathroom and started peeling my clothes off I looked at myself. Skin and bones…and this beard. I had lost thirty-three pounds.

I'm not equipped to evaluate warriors, but, from what I saw, those Marines were superb. I never saw a Marine officer or enlisted man who looked scared. That doesn't mean they weren't. Everybody was doing what had to be done. I never saw anybody smile and never heard any joking or clowning up there. But the Marines fought and fought well, and maintained discipline. They took care of the aid station and protected it. They supplied the vehicles when I needed them. They looked out for their wounded and brought all their wounded back.

There are few things in my life that I can feel as proud of as my service to this country in Korea with the 2nd Battalion, 5th Marines. I didn't like it one damn bit. I was there and luckily I survived. The Navy needed doctors and I happened to be one of them. I've been prouder of that than anything else I've ever done.

* * *

Bitter Cold and No Fires

In a letter to his father written immediately after the withdrawal to Hungnam, Dr. Chester Lessenden, Regimental Surgeon of the 5th Marines, recounts the stark terror of the hunted and the true horror that was Chosin.

December 11 or 12, 1950
Dearest Dad,

I haven't written for some time, but much has happened. I hardly know where to start.... On the night of Nov. 27 (Sunday) we arrived just north of Y-D-N (Yudam-ni) and just north of the 7th Marines position. That night we pitched our tents in the dark and prepared to do our usual work. About 11 pm all hell broke loose. We had heard an attack going on a mile north of us and had received about 40 casualties. We loaded all our vehicles and started them toward Hagaru [ri].

While they were gone, these Gooks started attacking *us*.[2] It seems there was a draw about 200 yards ahead and to our right. The Gooks used this draw to bypass our troops on the hills ahead and come down on us. Meanwhile, our vehicles returned with the news that there was a roadblock between us and Hagaru-ri. That was the start of it. We beat off the attack, all right, but the casualties continued to come in. At dawn on the 28th, our aid station moved a mile back and consolidated with the 7th Marines aid station. By the end of the day we were holding 400 patients and no place to put them. We got all the tents in both regiments (about 12) and took over four Gook houses. And still we had 100 or so. We put 18 inches of straw in this courtyard, put the patients in it, and covered it all with a big tarp. It was bitter cold, and no fires, of course, but I think those under the tarp spent the night better than anyone.

We stayed in this spot the 29th and got an air drop of tents (but no poles) stoves and blankets and stretchers. That night everyone was under cover and reasonably warm. We put straw on the tent floors and made them snug.

On the 30th word came we were to consolidate more and the aid station was to be taken in by the artillery. We made it but it took all day—move out the patients, take down the tents and haul them a couple of miles and put up the tent again and put the patients in it. I made the last trip on a helicopter. By this time we had about 600 patients. This night (the 30th) we all got a good night's sleep, the last for a while. I slept like a baby although the guns fired all night. They were the big 155s and they were firing in seven different directions. What I mean, we were surrounded.

The next day, Dec. 1, we got sudden word to pack all patients, burn our gear and prepare to get out of there.³ All non-litter casualties were to walk, as were we. So we did it. The frontlines were 20 yards from us by the time we got the last patient loaded and the gear fired. I never wanted to leave anyplace so much in my life, but those kids lying there on the stretchers never said a word, just awaited their turn.

In the fire I burned everything but my camera and the clothes I had on—my watch, a bottle of whiskey, a case of brandy, my little red leather suitcase and all my letters.

When the patients were loaded (it took practically every wheeled thing in both regiments and the artillery because by this time there were about 800 of them) we moved back 1½ miles and waited and waited and waited. I wish I could describe the scene to you but words fail me. The stream of vehicles laden with wounded, the crowd of men on the road, the smoke from burning gear and above all the terrible uncertainty of not knowing what was happening—no one knew and we all felt it. It's such an intangible thing but so real when it was happening—this "feeling."⁴

Anyway, we walked in circles all afternoon and night waiting for the word to move. It was another bitter cold night and these poor kids lying on litters on trucks and trailers and we didn't have enough stuff to keep them warm. Those that could walk we rotated through a Gook house all night (the MPs ran the civilians out). We used lots of morphine and the regimental chaplains (two of them) spent the night heating C rations in this Gook house for which I plan to write them up.⁵ They, the chaps, were so tired they could hardly stand, but they got everyone fed hot chow.

When the sun came up everything seemed a little better, but there had been lots of suffering during the night. Along in the middle of the day we got under weigh [*sic*]. We and our 800 charges slowly wound our way a mile or two when they stopped us in a field and lo and behold there were 50 or 60 more seriously wounded marines. Some way we got them aboard and again we waited for the convoy to move. Mind you, we could only move as far as the infantry could fight ahead of us opening the road. The harder the fight was the more people we had in our train.

Dr. [Howard] Greaves and I finally got these 60 aboard our sagging vehicles and we were exhausted. We located a hay stack and crapped out only we just about froze so we went into this gook house and it was so warm. We really soaked it up. So much so that our feet began to sweat. Eventually we got the word to move out. We'd move 50 yards and wait an hour. Dr. Greaves got sick so I put him in the last seat available and covered him up.

All that night we'd move and stop, move and stop. I sat down on the bumper of a truck and almost immediately went to sleep with my feet in the snow. That's when they froze. It was almost 24 hrs later that they began to hurt.

So that night and the next day we struggled up the mountain. I spent a good deal of the night kicking boys out of the snow so that they wouldn't freeze. Along in the afternoon we came to the top of the pass and horror of horrors we came to 50 or 60 more casualties. What to do—we resorted the ones we had, kicked those off who could possibly walk and put others on. We left there about dusk and breezed on to Hagaru. We simply staggered in.

When we arrived my good friend Ken Halloway gave me a shot of whiskey, a Nembutal and put me to bed but best of all he said, "We'll take over." It was just like taking off a tight girdle it felt so good to be out from under those 900 ineffectuals.

The next day was a mad house. Everyone wanted to get on a plane and be evacuated. The organization wasn't too good and many were evac[ed] because they could get to the airstrip. But by noon we had emerged from our stupor a little and got the situation under control. We sent out 1026 [casualties] the first [day] and 1350 the next. I dozed and ate and slept most of those two days and nursed my feet, and by the 3rd day I felt almost human.

We moved again late in the afternoon of the 3rd day and spent all night on the road again and arrived at Koto-ri about dark the following day (8 miles). But again we waited while the boys fought through....

On the 3rd day we started again at daylight down the *big* mountain. And this morning about 2 am we arrived here in Hamhung. The military people in our organization tell me we made military history in fighting our way out (through 10 divisions so scuttle butt has it). But I wouldn't know about that. I was concerned about my part of it—getting those patients through in as good a shape as possible...

Love,
Jack[6]

* * *

Silver Star Dentist

Morton Silver served briefly as an Army draftee during World War II before graduating from the New York University School of Dentistry at age twenty-two. "I felt I was much too young to go into practice and had no business skills. So I joined the Navy. I never had a day's training in the Army, Navy, or the Marine Corps. It seems impossible, but it was so. I just fell through the cracks. To serve with the Marine Corps you had to receive field medical training; I never received that, and I was strictly on my own."

In 1948, Dr. Silver was nevertheless assigned to the Fifth Battalion Landing Team of the 1st Marine Division. "We were going to have a parade one day. Everybody shined up their uniforms. The parade was to take place on Sunday. On

Saturday evening Korea was invaded. Immediately, we marched in that parade in battle gear—steel helmets, weapons. We had no intention of parading in battle gear, but Korea had just broken and the Marines wanted to make a show." He soon volunteered for Korean duty with the 5th Marines and saw action during the Inchon landing, Kimpo Airport, and the battle for Seoul. In the last days of November 1950, Dr. Silver and his comrades were fighting their way out of the Chinese trap at Chosin Reservoir.

I had a bag slung over my shoulder with a scalpel, a scissors, some forceps, and very little else. I don't think I ever used the forceps except once when I extracted an incisor on a Korean officer. I also carried morphine. The most important thing of all was that pair of scissors. I'm not joking. A scissors is most important. In fact, we didn't carry the scissors; we tied it around our waist so someone could never borrow it.

Once [Lt. Col. Ray] Murray caught me on the chow line without my carbine, and he demanded I carry a weapon. Every officer had to carry a weapon. So I got rid of the carbine and found a .45.

I didn't practice dentistry up there at Chosin. It was too serious a thing to worry about dentistry. Even so, we started getting men with fractured teeth. They were so hungry, and there was no way of heating up food. They would eat a cracker, open up a tin, and eat jelly. They also found Tootsie Rolls somewhere, a hell of a lot of Tootsie Rolls. When you put a frozen Tootsie Roll in your mouth it was like a rock. Yet the men wanted to get the taste, and they were smashing their teeth on them. If you had a tooth with a filling, forget it. The tooth was gone. Then the order went out: No more Tootsie Rolls.

It was getting colder and colder. One night, a jeep came in with its trailer. Inside were two wounded Chinese literally frozen into the trailer. We got them out and the colonel said to me, "Treat them." As we bandaged them, they were smiling and laughing. And then we interrogated them. We knew already that we were up against Chinese. We were sitting like a sore thumb up in the mountains. The road was a simple road—one-way. You couldn't get two trucks on that damn road. And we were stuck there.

While we were there, some of the Army troops came streaming through us. They were in complete disarray. I'll never forget the colonel saying, "Where is your doctor? Where's your wounded?"

And the answer was, "We couldn't do anything. We were under attack." And the colonel said, "Get them out of here. I don't want to talk to them [soldiers]." He wouldn't have anything to do with them because they abandoned their wounded.

On the retreat from the Chosin, we were walking along with a column of trucks. We tried to place a medical officer ahead, in the middle, and in the rear. I was somewhere near the middle. Soon we came across a kid lying by the side of the road. People were just walking by him because they couldn't stand to look. His whole head was a mass of blood—one huge mass of blood. I looked at him and walked on. I must have walked a hundred and fifty feet when I realized I just couldn't leave him there. So I went back. No one would go near him; he was so bloody.

I took huge packs of gauze and cotton and started wiping it away because it had congealed. And then I started laughing. He had a massive cut inside his mouth that was bleeding like crazy. The wound wasn't even worth a Purple Heart. He was young and healthy and because it was freezing cold, he wasn't bleeding to death. After I wiped out the blood, I jammed some gauze into his mouth and told him to hold onto it. Finally, he came out like a human being with a cut inside his mouth. Were we happy! I sent him on his way.

As we worked our way back from Hagaru [ri], we found some Marines lying in a field who needed care. Most of them were frozen with frostbite and couldn't walk. Then the rumor went around that we were pulling out. These kids were frightened out of their wits. They asked me, "Doctor, what's going to happen to us?"

After we issued weapons to those who could handle them, I went to the colonel and said, "Colonel, what are we going to do? The men are panic-stricken and we have no way of getting them out."

The colonel looked at me and said, "Silver, you go back and tell them that if we can't get them out we're not going out."

That night they warned us that the artillery was going to open up—155mm, 75mm cannon, everything. They aimed into the surrounding hills where the Chinese were. They fired every round we had all night long. In the morning, they blew up the guns and tore up the tires. Now we had about forty large trucks that once held the ammo for that artillery, and we piled the wounded from that field in them like cordwood. There was no other way of describing it. Two chaplains assisted me. They were wonderful. My back was so bad I looked like the letter C. I was so bent over I couldn't stand up anymore.

When the column stopped during the day, we started a fire under a fifty-five-gallon drum of water. We threw all the C-ration cans in there and when they were warm we tossed them into the truck. The men who were conscious and alive enough would open the cans and feed everybody.

The roads were highly crowned and covered with snow and packed almost like ice. And the column was moving very slowly. We were coming into Koto-ri. Chesty Puller's outfit had established a perimeter, and we were passing through it. I was pretty much near the end of the convoy when suddenly a truck filled with wounded went over the side. I saw a kid pinned underneath with the truck on top of him. Apparently his steel helmet was holding the truck up. I didn't know what the hell to do. A corpsman and I hauled the men out of the truck. There was primer cord in there and some kind of chlorine that was burning everybody. We took the men and dunked them in a nearby stream to get the stuff off. Even in that cold we found a stream with water running.

The question was how we were going to get this damn truck off the kid. I stood in the way and stopped the truck column. There weren't too many left, maybe a handful. A sergeant found a winch on one of them and we threw the cable over and hooked it onto the overturned truck. They moved it just enough to allow me to crawl underneath. I started pulling on the guy, the winch pulled the truck up a little more, and I yanked him free. The column then moved on.

The man had fractured legs. I took some stakes, put them between his legs, and wrapped them in a bundle. Fortunately, one of the chaplains came down the line and we were able to stop another truck. Even though all of them were filled to capacity with wounded, you could always shove somebody else in. There must have been eight or nine men from the vehicle that had gone over the side. We hauled them back onto the road and threw them onto the trucks. And that was the finish of the whole thing. I couldn't move anymore. They strapped me to the front fender of one of them, and that's how I rode into Koto-ri. I was young. I wasn't married. I was immortal. Furthermore, I wanted to win a medal. Of course, I didn't know I would get the Silver Star.

* * *

Corpsman Down

The fighting at Chosin Reservoir, which lasted two weeks, took a heavy toll on the Marines. They fell in droves from Chinese small arms and mortar fire or frostbite that left them helpless, unable to fight or walk without assistance. As in every war the Marines had ever fought in, hospital corpsmen shared their foxholes and risked their lives countless times a day. The corpsmen dragged Marines out of the line of fire, provided lifesaving aid, and tried to evacuate them to the rear. Second Lt. Joseph Owen, who commanded the 60mm mortars of Baker Company, 1st Battalion, 7th Marines, is very appreciative. "Our corpsmen were a very special breed of people. When they become corpsmen they become fearless. I never saw those guys falter. We had utmost confidence in them. They took care of some real tough cases—and multiple cases at one time. You'd get into a fire fight and suddenly have five or six guys down at once. And they often had to do instant triages—make a decision just like that. Which guy is he going to take care of first, and how much time he is going to spend with him? You'll never see any Marine who won't tell you that the greatest people in the world are his corpsmen."

The Chosin Reservoir campaign offered the hospital corpsman unique and unwelcome challenges. Bill Davis, one of Owen's beloved "docs," quickly learned to make do with what he had with him. "I carried a box of morphine syrettes next to my belly underneath all the clothing I had on. And I carried four of those syrettes in my mouth when we were going into action. That would keep them from freezing and keep them pliable."

Corpsmen were unarmed and conspicuous on the frontlines, which often meant that few of these brave men would return from the Chosin campaign unscathed or survive it at all. Bill Davis tells his story.

I remember Thanksgiving very well. Actually, it was the day after Thanksgiving. We went out on a patrol on Thanksgiving Day and got back very late at night. It was pitch dark, but the field kitchen was still there. And it was very, very cold. It was not twenty degrees below but ten degrees lower than that. The company came back so the field kitchen opened up to feed us. They had tin trays and they put the turkey and mashed potatoes on there and everything immediately froze. I couldn't even eat the mashed potatoes; they were hard. But we did eat the rest of the stuff even though it was cold because it was a meal.

Bear in mind it was darker than pitch. Joe Owen and I went over and found a jeep. We turned the lights on and sat on the hood eating so we could see what we were doing. When we did that we were illuminated. I recall a shot ricocheting off the jeep. There was a sniper somewhere firing at us, and Joe and I just sat there eating our meal and didn't even bat an eye at that sniper who really had poor aim.

We could see the Reservoir. It looked like a big ice skating rink. When we were in Hagaru [ri], it was right there. We walked on it in the course of moving up to some hill somewhere.

At that time we began moving in battalion as opposed to company because we had lost so many people. We were bivouacked on a hill, and Baker Company was sent out to make a reconnaissance on what we were going to do the next day. We went out into a valley. The Chinese were in the hills, and this was the first time they attacked us. They had mortar emplacements, had aimed them, and found out where they were going to land. Then they began throwing heavy automatic weapons and mortars at us.

We saw the enemy trying to attack down the side of a hill to overrun us, but they didn't make it because we had enough firepower to drive them back. The first line had weapons and the second and third line didn't. And the fourth line had weapons. So the second and third lines were attacking head-on and would pick up the weapons from the casualties in front of them. There were dead Chinese all over the place. They were armed with burp guns and even Thompson submachine guns. I don't know where they got those.

Eventually Charlie Company came up and helped us get out of there but we were there for hours under fire. I had five guys behind an outcropping of rock I had treated and was with them when somebody yelled, "Corpsman!"

So I got up to go and when I did, three of these guys got up to follow me. I turned around and said, "Stay there. I'm just going out to attend to another casualty. I'll be back." When I was in the process of hollering at them, a mortar shell went off right in front of me. All the shrapnel went through my open mouth and the side of my face, plus many other places on my body.

But there were more casualties and I had to take care of them. But before I could do that, I stopped first to put a bandage on. Now putting a bandage on inside the mouth is very difficult. I turned one of the bandages inside out, cut it, and then folded it in half so there would be gauze on both sides and stuffed it inside my mouth. That stopped some of the bleeding. My other wounds were in my chest, arms, and legs, but I was still functional. Then I took care of some casualties. The other guys, realizing I was in bad shape, helped out. By then Charlie Company showed up and some of their corpsmen took care of some of our people.

They took me back on a truck to Company C of the med battalion, and they put me next to the potbellied stove in the little dwelling they were using. After a while I told them they would have to move me because it was thawing out my feet and they were hurting like hell.

I was only there overnight, and the next morning an artillery observation airplane like a Piper Cub flew in and landed in the road beside the medical company. Then they loaded me aboard, but the door wouldn't close because the stretcher stuck out. The plane had a black Army pilot. I'd never seen a black Army pilot before. It didn't matter to me. He was going to get me the hell out of there. They ended up tying the door to the end of the stretcher so it wouldn't flap around. He took off from the road and flew me back to a MASH unit because they had oral surgeons there.

That flight was colder than hell! The wind was blowing right in through the open door. Even though he wasn't flying very high, the ground temperature was thirty below zero! The flight was less than thirty minutes long, and I ended up very close to Hamhung.

They debrided the wound and took out lots of metal that was in my mouth and did some bandaging. They were also going to do some surgery to keep the facial tissue together. I had a hole in the roof of my mouth that went up into my sinus on the left side.

From there I went to the Fukuoka Army Hospital. Fortunately, I was only there three days before they flew me to Yokosuka and things got back to normal.

Actually it wasn't normal because there were twenty-six hundred patients there. These were the casualties from the Chosin Reservoir. My place in the hospital was in the corpsmen's quarters. The nurses' quarters was a ward and the hospital was a ward. The passageways were a ward. Even the auditorium was filled with patients. Prior to evacuation back to the states, my bed was on the stage of the auditorium. The staff lived in the caves which the Japanese had built around the hospital. They cared for me very well as they did for all casualties in what was a crowded and confusing environment.

The same great care was duplicated as I was returned to the States and ultimately to the Philadelphia Naval Hospital. They didn't do anything for my frostbite at Yokosuka, but did so when I got back to Philadelphia Naval Hospital, where I stayed for six months. I was on an ear, nose, and throat ward right next door to a ward where they had forty-two patients. At least forty of those were frostbite patients. There were six different types of treatment going on at the same time. They didn't know how to treat them. You would find a guy in a bed with a heat cradle over the top of his feet, with a light in there to warm them. You would go down two beds and there was a guy with an icepack on his feet. Two more beds down you'd see a patient with nothing but a fan blowing on his feet. It was hit and miss.

I didn't get any treatment for my frostbite because mine didn't bother me. It bothered me in later years, though. I lost my toe nails and to this day they keep falling off. I still had feeling in my feet so I wasn't a real candidate for treatment.

I still have shrapnel in my chest. It turned out that a fragment about the size of my thumbnail had worked its way down behind the sternum, where it resides to this day. Fortunately, it's covered in scar tissue so it doesn't move, and hasn't since 1951.

I still have five pieces in my face. They took the tissue from the right side of the roof of my mouth and flopped it over to the left side of my mouth where this big hole was. And that's how they closed up the hole. Then they made me a plastic denture—a guard—which I wore all the time until the flap began to heal and was strong enough. I was on a liquid diet for four months! Back in 1951, the normal liquid diet was Jello, soup, and milkshakes, period. After that I ended up weighing eighty-five pounds.

The fragments in my face don't bother me. I had some in my leg and arm that came out by working their way to the surface. We just plucked them out. I should say that this mouth wound took out the whole left inside of my face. It took the gum, the bone, and the teeth so there was just a great big hole there. Before I got out of the Philadelphia Naval Hospital, they made a prosthesis for me but I couldn't eat on that side. They couldn't replace the gum or bone. In fact, it was seventeen years later, in 1967, that an oral surgeon at Bethesda [National Naval Medical Center] did a bone and tissue transplant to give me gum and bone in the left side of my mouth.

* * *

Circling the Wagons

Like Bill Davis, the corpsman who took care of his men, 2nd Lt. Joe Owen's appreciation of Navy medicine is genuine and comes from firsthand experience.

We were like a reinforced rifle platoon and by that time down to about fifty people. We were on a company-sized patrol on 27 November, and the Chinese surrounded us about five miles from the battalion perimeter. We just circled the wagons and were waiting for them to come at us that night. We were running out of ammo. [Edmond] Mickens and Bill Davis formed their own temporary aid station in the middle of our perimeter with the Chinese shooting in at us.

Mickens got it fairly early. They had him stretched out. Bill Davis was trying to take care of him. One of my men directed a stretcher detail and he was going all over the place picking up bodies. They took them to where Davis was treating the wounded. We lost two platoon sergeants, and the skipper got hit through the mouth. Bill Davis was leading a walking wounded guy and was trying to get him over to where the stretchers were. As he did so, he took a piece of shrapnel through the mouth and couldn't talk. He tried to keep working but after a while he couldn't and they put him down. I don't know whether anybody took care of the wounded after that.

I remember one morning after we had gotten into Hagaru [ri], we got a replacement corpsman. The gunny told him, "Just stick by me and then when you hear a guy start yelling 'corpsman,' you go to where they're yelling 'corpsman.'" That was that guy's indoctrination because we started moving out right away.

On the 8th of December, we had the point for the division. We were down to about 30 men of our original 215 plus maybe another 100 replacements who had come to us over two campaigns. Our skipper had just been killed. There were three lieutenants left. [1st Lt. Chew-Een] Lee took over. He got hit in twenty minutes. The Chinese were up on a hill and we had to make a frontal assault on them. I was leading the assault. For a while we had a tank but that pulled off. I had [Pfc. Attilio] Lupacchini with me and the two of us were forward. Lupacchini was right next to me and he went down fast. And then I got nailed. A couple of Gooks popped up from behind a hill a little ways from me. One had a rifle, the other a burp gun. The guy with the rifle got me in my left side, the burp gunner got me on the right side. I went down in the snow. I think I got two or three rounds from the burp gun; I'm not sure. But it blew out my elbow and most of the nerves. The pain was awful. I was also spitting blood all over the place. Later I found out that when the bullet entered my upper left shoulder and came out my back, it knocked off part of the scapular bone. In doing so, it nicked my lung. That's why a lot of people thought I was dead when they saw me lying beside the road. The whole front of me was covered with blood.

[Cpl. Eugene M.] Morrisroe was coming up right behind me and he saw those Chinese. He shot the Chinese rifleman with his M1 and somebody else got the burp gunner, perhaps [Cpl. Merwin] Perkins. When Morrisroe got up to where the dead Chinese rifleman was, he saw him holding a new clip of .25 caliber ammo in his hand. He was about to reload because the round he got me with was the last one in the clip [in his rifle]. As he went by, Morrisroe took that fresh clip of ammo from the Chinese and saved it as a souvenir. Many years later, he gave it to me and I have it framed on my wall.

After I got shot, the corpsman who got to me was a replacement who had just joined us that day. I don't know who he was. He was the only one with us who had a clear, shaven face and a clean parka. He stood out because he was so new. He didn't know what the hell was going on.

The fire was very heavy yet this kid came up about a hundred yards, under that fire, across a snowy hill to get to me. Then he threw himself down beside me. Bullets were whizzing just a few inches overhead. As he lay beside me, I yelled at him to give me some morphine and he said he couldn't. "I can't, sir. It's frozen."

And then I really took off at him. "Put it in your mouth and keep it liquid. Don't you boots know anything?" Then I realized this kid has come up under fire to save my life, and I'm chewing him out.

After a while the morphine melted and he gave me the jab. I'll never forget chewing him out after what he had just done. I was ashamed of myself. I'd give anything to find that lad and thank him. Of the twenty-seven people who survived our company, not one of them knows what happened to that corpsman. He was the second one we had in two days. The first had been killed the previous day, and no one even knew who he was.

There was a lot of confusion about how I got down off the hill. What we did with casualties was to open up a poncho or shelter half and put the guy on it. Then we slid him down on the snow. That saved a four-man carry. Two or three guys claimed to have taken me down and put me in a ditch.

By this time I was in and out of it with the morphine. I woke up once and a huge tank was chuffing away. I wondered if he knew I was there and was afraid he'd run over me.

Anyway, I was down in the ditch and coming in and out of consciousness. I had sent [Cpl. Robert] Kelly, my runner, back earlier to take what was left of our 60s [mortars]. He came down the road and saw me there. I guess there were a lot of casualties around. A crackerbox ambulance was sitting on the road with a couple of corpsmen in it getting warm. You couldn't blame them for that. They'd been working hard that day. Kelly went up and told them he had a bad casualty. When the corpsmen gave him a hard time, Kelly shoved his carbine into the ambulance. That convinced them to load me aboard. The ambulance held four. I remember one guy screaming for morphine and another guy telling him to quit his bitchin'. I wanted some morphine, too, but the corpsman told me he couldn't give me any until we got back to the aid station.

I remember being carried into the aid station, a huge canvas affair with bright lights. People began stripping and doing things to me. I woke up a couple of times with guys moaning. The corpsmen were wearing scarves around their faces. They were all in their parkas, all wrapped up. It was cold. I remember looking up and seeing plasma and wondering if it was going to freeze.

I ended up in an Army field hospital in an old schoolhouse. When I woke up, I saw high windows and then this beautiful, beautiful woman only inches from my face. She looked like an Irish colleen with black hair and blue eyes. I thought I was dead and in heaven, and I figured she was an angel. My first thought was, "I made it." I never thought *I* would make it to heaven. Then I wondered how my wife Dorothy would find out I was dead.

It turned out she was checking my vital signs. After that, two giant black guys carried me on a stretcher to a plane. One of them kept telling me, "You're going to be all right, man. You're going to be all right now." He said, "The Air Force takes care of you now." So they flew me out of Korea.

When I woke up, it was like a nightmare. Brueghel could have painted this scene. It was a big, open room like a gymnasium with cots all over the place and people moaning and screaming. I noticed that the blankets were brown, and then I heard someone yelling, "Medic!" It was an Army hospital. At that time, the Army had not performed well up where we were fighting and I had little respect for them. I guess that translated into my thinking. I was indignant that I was in an Army hospital. I yelled out for a corpsman. I didn't want some medic taking care of me. I wanted a corpsman.

I was only in that Army hospital at Otsu for a day or so. And when I woke up, I was being pushed into the junior officers' ward at the naval hospital in Yokosuka. That's a scene that should be captured. All the passageways there at Yokosuka were lined with cots. There were guys sitting or smoking or walking around. Those were mainly the walking wounded. Guys badly wounded like me were in rooms in beds. It was the same in the junior officers' ward. A nurse came in. We called her "Nurse Gunny." She was some tough cookie, but I love her to this day.

When they brought me to Yokosuka, I learned that I also had frostbite. I hadn't realized that. I must have gotten it after I was wounded and lying in the ditch. Even though it was a mild case, it upset me greatly. To me, avoiding frostbite was a function of discipline. You could always hear the NCOs and junior officers yelling,

"Keep your toes moving." When you're pinned down, you just had to remember to keep the pieces moving. And I hadn't done that after I got wounded. I do remember waking up with that tank over my head and remembering to wiggle my toes. I had the thought, "Jeez, an officer getting frostbite."

The day after I got to Yokosuka, Japanese orderlies took me through innumerable passageways into an examining room. I was just coming out of a haze and saw three Navy doctors. They were looking at a light board with x-rays on it. I heard one say, "We can't do anything with this arm."

Then a big Navy captain said, "Gentlemen, I guess the only thing we can do is amputate."

And I thought, "Some poor bastard is going to get something amputated. I lifted my head up a little bit to see what poor bastard was going to have something cut off. And then I realized that I was alone. Suddenly it dawned that they were talking about me! When I heard him say "amputate," I sat up as far as I could and said, "Fuck you! You're not amputatin' anything off me." As you know, you don't say that to a Navy captain.

He came over and said, "Lieutenant, you just have to face facts and realize that there's not much we can do."

I said, "I've got to get back to my troops. I can't get back to my troops if I don't have an arm." Getting back to my troops was always in my head.

He patted me a few times and then turned to the other two doctors and said, "Gentlemen, with this kind of spirit, let's see what happens. We've got enough work here. If they want to take it off back in the States . . . let's see if they'll work with him." So they all nodded their heads and that's why they didn't cut my arm off.

What got him was what I said about getting back to my troops. That was just as sincere as any thought I've ever had in my life. All I could think of was, "They need me." And I couldn't go back if I didn't have my arm.

I remember some time after that when a doctor came in to check my arm. They had me in a half cast by that time. It was awful; I couldn't even look at it. I asked what he thought. He said, "I'm not the guy you should ask. I'm only here to get it cleaned up and make sure you don't have any infection spreading."

I said, "Well, tell me what's going to happen? When are we gonna start getting this thing going?"

He said, "You want to talk to a nerve man or a bone doctor."

"But I'm talking to you."

He said, "This isn't my line."

"What's your line?"

He said, "I'm a pediatrician."

"What the hell are you doing here?"

He said, "That's what I'd like to know."

A couple of weeks before he was probably taking care of little babies. Now he was taking care of big babies. He was one of the few people I ran into in that whole hospitalwho didn't seem to put himself out for you. He was feeling sorry for himself. It seems that some of those doctors had been yanked right out of wherever they were.

After that, the nurses and corpsmen encouraged me to eat and do things. The nurses were so kind. The walking wounded wanted to get back to Korea. Most of us were regulars. The problem the nurses and doctors had there was trying to keep these guys subdued because all they wanted to do was get back on the line.

When I left Yokosuka, I went out on a gurney, and they stopped me at the nurses' station. "Nurse Gunny" came out, held my hand, and kissed me. And they were all like that. They were beautiful to us. And the corpsmen. I had problems with some of them back in the States but those corpsmen at Yokosuka were great.

We got to the Army hospital at Tripler and that was like paradise. It was a beautiful place. By this time I was half-casted. There was nothing medically significant at Tripler except they were so good to us. They kept bringing us fruit, flowers. The windows were open and I could look out over the ocean.

I ended up at the naval hospital in St. Albans [New York]. I believe a Capt. James, who I think was a neurosurgeon, came into my room and gave me an extensive examination. I had a severed ulnar nerve. The doctors in the x-ray room said it looked to them like a bombed-out railroad yard with the tracks all shot up. Dr. James prodded me with pins and I couldn't feel anything. He could have been jumping up and down on my arm for all I knew. It had no feeling whatsoever. He told me that I would have to learn to do things with my left hand and start adjusting to a new way of doing things. At that time, I thought I would be going back to duty. I just knew something was going to bring this arm back.

A few days later there was a flag inspection and the admiral came in with a huge staff and Capt. James. I happened to be sitting on my sack at that time writing a letter. Capt. James pointed that out to the admiral. "Just look at the spirit of these Marines. I just talked to him the other day about learning how to do things with his other hand."

And the admiral said, "Do you mind if I take a look at what you're writing, lieutenant?" So he saw my handwriting and said, "You're off to a very good start." I didn't have the heart to tell him I was left-handed, and he never found out.

My arm never came back so I could go to full duty, or any duty at all. When I finally realized I was going to have an arm that would not function, I was prepared for it and didn't whine or wonder how I was going to live with a disability when I got out.

I'd get terribly frustrated learning to cut meat and had the corpsman do it for me. And that was terrible having to have someone do that for me. For a long time afterward, I didn't go to restaurants because I'd have to ask the waiter to have my meat cut.

I was in the hospital a year and half and, by the time I got out, I was acclimated to what I had. Maybe, too, there were guys a lot worse than I was. Nobody sat around saying, "I feel sorry for you" or "You've got it tough." There was no quarter given. That was the great thing about it.

While I was at St. Albans, I had a series of operations—exploratories and patching the bones together, and fixing the nerves. They also took me to Columbia Presbyterian Hospital. One of the leading hand specialists in the world, a Dr. Carroll, did a lot of work on me. After I was surveyed out of the Marine Corps, I kept exercising and, a couple of years later, my arm started to improve drastically. They had put me on a regimen of constant exercise when I was in the hospital and that stayed with me. I always carried a little rubber ball around and squeezed it. I began to get feeling in my hand and noticed I could make some movements.

I was in New York on business once—about 1954—and went to the Naval Hospital and asked them to take a look. I went back in for two operations and there was a drastic improvement in my hand. Now you can see I have a pretty good hand! It became a challenge for me to do things and I give the credit to those people who never, ever gave me the soft treatment. I think they sensed that a guy like me needed tough treatment. When I think of my time in naval hospitals, I think of how fortunate I was. As long as I had to get shot, thank God I had the naval hospitals to take care of me.

The 7.62mm burp gun slugs that hit Owen during the withdrawal from Koto-ri caused a compound comminuted fracture of his right ulna and radius at the elbow joint resulting in an ulnar and median nerve injury. The .25 caliber (6.5mm) rifle bullet, fired from a World War II Japanese rifle, entered above his left shoulder and exited his chest. This produced a compound comminuted fracture of the left scapula, a far less serious wound.

* * *

Flight Nurse Under Fire

Lillian Keil was a veteran Air Force flight nurse, having earned four Battle Stars for her service in Europe during World War II—Normandy, the Battle of the Bulge, northern France, and the Rhineland. When the Korean War broke out, she was working as a stewardess for United Airlines based in San Francisco. In June 1950, 1st Lt. Keil quit United and picked up where she left off, flying to Tokyo as an Air Force flight nurse. Although headquartered in Japan, her beat was everywhere that Air Force evacuation aircraft flew in Korea.

Her first evac flights took place during the Inchon-Seoul operations in September 1950. As the Chosin drama unfolded and casualties mounted, Air Force and Marine aircraft stood by awaiting the completion of the primitive landing strip at the besieged village of Hagaru-ri. To build this airstrip, Marine Corps engineers gouged the frozen earth using high explosives and bulldozers with steel teeth welded to their blades. When this herculean task was completed, Air Force C-47s of the Combat Cargo Command's 801st Squadron—the "Kyushu Gypsies"—and several Marine R4Ds began unloading precious supplies and evacuating the most seriously wounded and frostbitten cases. By 6 December, more than four thousand men had been evacuated from Hagaru-ri's frozen airstrip. And all these feats of construction and evacuation were accomplished under fire; the Chinese occupied the hills just beyond the Marines' perimeter. Flight nurse Keil recalls the vivid memories.

Hagaru [ri] was surrounded on three sides by mountains, and it depended upon the weather as to what approach we could make. When we got there, we would unload whatever we had brought in for the troops—military supplies, gasoline, oil, rations, clothing, shells—whatever the fighting man needed. Air-evac always carried military supplies to the forward areas. On some flights the whole airplane was full of five-gallon cans of gasoline. And there were a lot of times we also carried as many fifty-gallon oil drums as we could get on the airplane. The little port holes had to be left open [because of the fumes]. If they were closed, and there was a spark, the gasoline would explode, and everybody would be lost.

There was no doctor aboard our flights, only a medical technician and a flight nurse. The patients were in critical situations, and we had to be very careful. The planes weren't pressurized. We didn't maintain a high altitude because the altitude affected the head cases.

We flight nurses carried a blanket bag, a duffel bag about two feet across and about two and a half feet long. We also had blankets. There were several times when I had a flight suit made of lamb's wool inside, and pants. I covered the patients who were shivering with the cold with my flight jacket or took off my flight pants and put those over them.

On most flights into Hagaru [ri] we heard the gunfire. There was only one approach we could make. It was touch-and-go for the pilots if the weather was bad. Fortunately, I never saw bullets flying through the plane, but I heard the rumble [of artillery].

There was one flight I remember very well. Everybody was scared. We didn't even know whether or not we would be able to get in because of the weather. It was really touch-and-go and kind of difficult for the pilots because it was their first trip in. I know that when we landed, we landed very short and they wouldn't let me out of the plane. We picked up our patients and then took off as soon as we were loaded.

Whenever the door was open, I could see out. There was nothing but snow and slush. GIs were running around, and military equipment was being off-loaded. There was a lot of frantic work being accomplished in order to get the plane off again. As the plane was unloaded we would take down the litter straps and get ready to take aboard whatever patients they had for us. We could accommodate twenty-four litter patients.

A corpsman would set up the ramp and then carry the wounded aboard on a stretcher. I had an extra stretcher handy, and would have the corpsman transfer the patient to the clean stretcher. Then, from the doorway, we would shake out the old stretcher and blankets and put the patient back on it. Some of them had a lot of dirt under their necks; some didn't have many clothes on, just a blanket. But that little thing we did was something they really appreciated.

It was horrible. Some of the boys were wet, others were in great pain. And others were shivering from the cold. There was one trip I remember when the boys came aboard in just their stocking feet. These fellows left their shoes behind for those who needed them badly. And it was so cold.

The guys were very happy to see me. Even as bad as everything was, they would smile and say, "It's so wonderful to see an American woman." It made me feel good. We worked hard, but if a wounded GI smiled at us, it was a beautiful sight. Let me put it this way. When you got a load of patients, it didn't matter who they were or what their wounds. You had a load of wounded personnel who were in pain. Even so, they were happy. All of a sudden it was, "Oh, we're going home. We are getting out of here."

As soon as the plane was loaded we took off. Then another plane, right behind us, landed as we took off and picked up more patients. Right away, the most important thing was to get the men into position on the airplane. We couldn't do much about treating them until we got the door closed and started looking around to see who needed help the most. Most of them would have had medic first aid. The corpsmen would have put an "MS" on the foreheads of the patients to let us know that they had received morphine. If a patient had had a gunshot wound in the thigh, for example, the clothing would be torn at that point so that the corpsman could get to the wound. It was bloody, muddy, dirty, smelly, everything. But you just had to ignore that and check the bandages to see if the wound was bleeding. There was not much more we could do but provide the quick aids and whatever the person needed.

We couldn't wash their wounds but we did have sterile saline solution. If there was a great deal of bleeding and there was a lot of dirt in the wound, we got our sponges and used the saline. Sometimes we just dropped a saline pad on top of the wound after I cleansed it. But most of that work had already been done. Many of these boys were going to rear echelons and MASH hospitals to have surgery.

There was very little we could do for the frostbite patients except keep them warm. With frostbite, you'd think the patient would be in a lot of pain but that wasn't the case. We simply covered them with blankets.

From Hagaru [ri] we flew back to the first airfield with facilities for medical care or surgery. We left those patients there and then went back to get more. If that airfield was already filled to capacity with wounded, we went to another facility. Maybe in a day or so, depending upon our schedule, we went back to one of these airfields, picked up patients, and brought them to Japan.

A few patients stand out in my mind. I remember one boy who had gotten frostbite and now had black stumps for fingers. Another, whose face was practically eliminated, nevertheless asked for a pencil and paper. I have that paper in front of me right now. I've saved it all these years. He wrote, "Do you think I will live? Will I get to go home? When we get to the hospital please tell them to...." He overwrote the first words and I can't make them out.

Well, here it is fifty years later and I sometimes ask myself if I was really there. Occasionally I feel that I have probably seen it all in a movie. Nevertheless, I really enjoyed putting my whole heart into my work. I thought it was the most wonderful thing to be where I was, flying and taking care of all those boys.

Notes
[1]Bullae are liquid-filled, and in this case, frozen elevations on the skin.

[2]According to Corpsman Herbert Renner, "The enemy—North Korean and Chinese troops–were called 'Gooks' (or 'Luke the Gook') collectively, along with anyone else who supported their side, including the Russians or any other communists. The word 'Gook' had no ethnic origin, was coined long before ethnic correctness was in vogue, and was not meant to be denigrating to those to which it was directed. It was entirely a military word disassociated with civilian life invented by warriors who had to fight the enemy."

[3]Lessenden's wife Edith recalls her late husband elaborating on the destruction of gear. "They were to destroy everything, except for small items they could put in a pocket or hang around their necks. They built a big bonfire, well doused with gasoline and oil and threw everything on it. For example, Chet threw in his personal possessions, his leather suitcase, and his Bausch and Lomb binoculars, which had been my Christmas gift the previous year, and a bundle of my letters. The only things he kept were his surgeon's tools, packaged in a Marine-green canvas roll-up, the medical supply of blood, which he wore next to his skin to keep it from freezing, his 35mm camera, and a few rolls of film."

[4]Edith Lessenden continues, "All during the retreat down the mountain was the ubiquitous background growl of heavy engines of ambulances, jeeps, etc. For months after returning home, Chet got a rush of adrenaline every time he heard the sound of a heavy engine. He used to joke about it, saying he was just like Pavlov's dog."

[5]Lt. Col., now Maj. Gen. Ray Murray (retired), commanding officer of the 5th Marines, was consumed with the responsibility of leading his troops out of the Chosin trap. Nevertheless, he vividly recalls this incident. "He [Lessenden] was in a hut and there was a huge pot of some kind that belonged to the people who lived there. They built a fire under it and were thawing C-rations in it to give to the wounded. He and the other doctors worked day and night to take care of these people. I don't know when they slept."

[6]Lessenden was "Les" to his regimental commander, "Chet" to his wife, and "Jack" to his father.

4

Yokosuka

*T*he land-based Navy medical treatment facility closest to the Korean fighting was an old Japanese hospital on the Yokosuka Naval Base. The former dispensary had been occupied by U.S. forces since World War II. In August 1950, two months after the outbreak of the war, Naval Hospital Yokosuka was officially established and shortly expanded to accommodate 5,000 patients. On 6 and 7 December, 2,022 patients were admitted, most of them casualties of the Chosin Reservoir campaign from the past two weeks. Many were suffering from frostbite. To accommodate the influx, double and, in some places, triple-decker bunks replaced regular hospital beds. As the war dragged on, Yokosuka's medical staff treated and returned many Marines and sailors to their units. For many others requiring more specialized care and long recuperation, Yokosuka was but a way station in the chain of evacuation back to military hospitals in the continental United States.

* * *

Temporary Additional Duty

Dr. Robert P. Dobbie was the only son of a surgeon who had served in World War I as an army officer. He entered the University of Michigan for undergraduate study in 1941 and joined the Navy V-1 program the following year.[1] He then became part of V-12, the Navy's program for advanced medical school education, and received his degree at the end of 1946.

With demobilization, Dobbie was discharged, as were many other young physicians who had received their medical education under V-12. The following year, the Navy offered him a commission as a lieutenant (j.g.) while allowing him to finish his surgical residency. In July 1950, Dobbie was ordered to active duty and reported to Naval Hospital Oakland, California, for what was to be a twenty-four-hour interlude. He was soon on his way to Yokosuka, Japan, to join Surgical Team Number Eight. Until the team's services were required, its members were assigned Temporary Additional Duty, helping to treat the many casualties flooding in from the Korean front.

I arrived in Yokosuka sometime in September of 1950 just as the Inchon landing was occurring. The Yokosuka Naval Hospital was an old Japanese naval hospital, which had been, until six weeks previously, a relatively small dispensary with most of the wards closed because they were not needed. Within six weeks this dispensary was expanded from maybe 20 or 30 beds to about 150 beds with continuing expansion going on from the time I arrived. I believe the size of the hospital ultimately reached 500 or 600 beds, and at the time of the evacuation of the Marines from the Chosin Reservoir we had responsibility for over 5,000 patients. Not all of them—as a matter of fact, very few of them—could be taken care of in the hospital because it wasn't that big and the majority of the casualties were frostbite casualties with toes and fingers badly frostbitten.

Otherwise the Marines were reasonably healthy so we kept them in old Japanese barracks in bunk beds that were four or five tiers high. We made rounds rather hastily, looking at their fingers and toes on a twice-a-day basis. Evacuation of these frostbitten men was accomplished back to either Hawaii or all the way back to the United States over a period of the next four to six weeks.

This period of frostbite in the Chosin Reservoir took place in late November and early December of 1950. When I arrived in Yokosuka, I was assigned to Surgical Team Number Eight. The team was then functioning in temporary duty capacity at the Yokosuka Naval Hospital where I was assigned to a combined neurosurgical and urology ward where the paraplegics and urologic cases were handled.

The wounded arrived daily at the train station at Yokosuka and were transferred by ambulance to the hospital. And as I said, the hospital was expanding almost on a daily basis, and we were receiving large numbers of severely wounded Marines within 24 to 48 hours of their having been wounded, which to me seemed quite remarkable.

Most were pretty well stabilized by the time they got to us, and our job was more definitive surgical repair. We all worked very hard and tried to keep control of the huge numbers of patients. All the time, more and more medical officers and nurses were arriving to help out so that we had a pretty reasonable balance in terms of numbers of patients for whom we were responsible and medical personnel— corpsmen, nurses, and physicians—to take care of them.

Because paraplegic patients frequently have urologic problems, it was decided that the paraplegics would all be on the urology ward. We had some 20 or 30 paraplegic patients and perhaps some 20 or 30 urology patients. About a third— maybe 10 or possibly 15—of the urology patients simply had severe cases of gonorrhea and as such were being treated on the urology service.

One day the Secretary of the Navy [Francis P. Matthews] came by wanting to give Purple Heart medals to some severely wounded Marines. And because Marines with paraplegia were considered to be severely wounded, he started at one end of the paraplegic ward and passed out Purple Hearts to all the patients. Unfortunately, he did not know and understand that patients with simple gonorrhea were also on the ward. So, as he continued down the line, he gave Purple Hearts to Marines who were there only because they had contracted gonorrhea while on liberty. None of the medical officers or other medical personnel were able to get to him in time, and we all felt a little embarrassed. I guess we were afraid to tell him what he had just done.

On a happier note, sometime in the early fall of 1950, Bob Hope visited the hospital. Because he wanted to see severely injured people, he came to our ward. After being told that not all the patients on the ward were severely wounded, he confined his visit to the paraplegics and spent between five and 10 minutes with each one. A member of his staff took a picture of him with each patient.

I remember one in particular. Hope asked him where he was from and the man said he was from Seattle. Hope then said that as soon as he left Japan he was going to Seattle to put on a show. He asked for the address of the man's parents and said he would drop in on them and let them know that he had seen their son and that he was doing reasonably well, all things considered.

I really thought this was a bunch of baloney and never really believed that he would take the time to look up this kid's folks. But three weeks later he got a letter from his parents explaining that Bob Hope had not only called but had insisted on taking them out to dinner. I was tremendously impressed. Needless to say, Bob Hope will remain forever one of my favorite heroes from the Korean or any other war.

Though we were confronted with many grisly wounds, I remember the unusual ones that perhaps were not quite so grisly. One was a soldier who had stuck his head over a trench and had a sniper catch him right between the eyes. The bullet went through his skull and out the back of his head. But for a fingertip-sized hole in his forehead and a much bigger hole in the back of his skull, he healed very nicely. His head x-ray showed a few little metallic fragments along the midline course of the bullet path as it passed cleanly through his head from front to back without any neurologic injury. The tragic part of the story was that the Army was so desperate that anybody who was felt to be reasonably able and with healing wounds was required to be sent back to his unit.

We kept this soldier for ten days, eight days beyond the time when he was well enough to go back to duty, simply because we didn't have the heart to send him back to his unit. Nevertheless, we were ultimately required to send him back and we did.

Another wound I recall was also a head wound. In this case, the bullet had gone through the front lip of the man's helmet, impacted on his skull, burrowed 270 degrees around his skull, and exited without ever penetrating. Apparently the steel of the helmet had taken enough of the sting off the bullet and, because it was a tangential blow, the bullet ran along the skull between the scalp and the skull three-quarters of the way around his head before it exited.

Yet another wound was to a Marine who had been charging up a hill yelling with his mouth open. He suddenly felt a stinging sensation at the base of his tongue. As he reached his hand around, he felt a bloody hole in the back of his head. This evidence convinced him that he was going to die. So he simply lay down as the battle raged on over him for perhaps a half hour. When it ended, he recalled lying there for about another hour. Then, because he hadn't died, he got up and walked to the aid station, still not believing he was alive. When he reached us, we found a simple through and through wound. The bullet had passed across the base of his tongue, and he had an exit wound at the base of his skull which healed satisfactorily. He also had to return to duty, but was incredulous that he had survived such a potentially devastating wound.

And yet, another experience. A young Marine was charging up a hill with a BAR, [Browning Automatic Rifle], which he was holding at port arms. He was passing a tree when a Chinese soldier jumped out and, from five yards away, sprayed him with a Thompson submachine gun. As the gun rose from the recoil, four bullets struck the stock of his BAR which was being held across his abdomen. The stock took the major impact of the four .45 caliber slugs but splinters from the back of the stock were driven into the Marine's abdomen. We had to operate on him to be sure those splinters were removed and that none of them had penetrated any vital organs, which they had not. It was obvious that the stock of his weapon had saved him from serious injury.

* * *

"Ward Victor"

Marilyn Ewing Affleck was carrying on the family tradition when she decided to become a nurse. In fact, the West Virginia native attended the same nursing school in East Liverpool, Ohio, where her mother had graduated in 1919. When Ewing joined the Navy in 1948, she went to the training center at Great Lakes, Illinois, to learn the basics of Navy life—marching and how to wear the uniform.

She was on the staff of Naval Hospital Camp Pendleton, California, working on the dependents' ward when the war broke out in Korea. Shortly thereafter, news arrived that the Marine husband of one of her civilian colleagues had been killed in action. "That was our first real thought of what was going on over there. Then we saw boys going on the buses. They would throw their letters out and ask us if we would mail them. They left Pendleton by the busloads." Ewing, too, was soon on her way to the Far East. Her new assignment was Naval Hospital Yokosuka, Japan.

I was excited. We were finally going to do something. We began getting all the shots we needed, then packed up all our gear and left for San Diego. From there we flew to San Francisco, stayed for two or three days, and then went to Seattle. From there we flew to Alaska, Shemya, and then Tokyo. The whole trip probably took five days. We got in late at night or very early in the morning, and they put us in dependents' housing. We had to get up and be in the chief nurse's office by eight. We were tired. I remember leaning up against the wall falling asleep.

Yokosuka was a Japanese hospital that had been converted with long rows of wards on either side. There were brick and cement type corridors. It was a little rustic but they did everything they could to make it good for us. We didn't have any complaints about that. I worked on "Ward Victor."

The routine was pretty much like in any other hospital. The first thing you did in the morning was to get your report from the night nurse and then make your rounds checking all the patients. Then the corpsmen would go around with the medicines. When the doctors arrived, we made doctors' rounds. Then we did dressing changes. The chow cart then came along and anybody who could walk went to get their chow. We took the food to the others.

We did the usual day of patient care. We rubbed their backs and made sure they turned over every two hours. And we turned them if they couldn't do it on their own. That was the way it was.

It seemed like we all worked together—nurses and corpsmen. We knew that we [the nurses] had to take care of the keys for the narcotics and make sure the medications were given. But if a patient wanted a back rub or the urinal or something, you didn't tell a corpsman to go get it. You'd go get it yourself. No one waited for corpsmen to do everything. You couldn't. They were just as busy as we were.

There were a lot of young men in the hospital, three high in some bunks on our wards. The ones who could move were on the top bunk and the one ones who couldn't were on the bottom bunk where we could handle them.

I was on orthopedics. Some of the other wards had VD patients and some cared for patients without arms. There was also an OB/dependent ward where I worked for a while, and an officers' ward. All the wards were all spread out and were full.

I think most of the patients from the Chosin got there before we arrived in December, maybe a week before Christmas. We soaked their feet in a basin of warm water and used our bandage scissors to scrape the black crud, calluses, and stuff off their feet. It was difficult. Some of them hadn't had a bath in weeks. These weren't frostbite cases. Those patients were on a different ward.

We had two young Marines on our ward. One had been hit by a land mine and his buddy went out to get him. The first one lost a leg. And the other lost the opposite leg. You should have seen the two of them carry on. They would get together, hop, and walk arm in arm. They really adjusted well at our place.

Once I substituted on a ward where there was a Marine who lost both hands. It was near Christmas. The Salvation Army had sent packages, and we were going around putting them on the patients' bedside tables. We didn't wake them up to say "Merry Christmas" unless we saw that they were awake. I felt really bad and didn't want to wish Merry Christmas to the young man missing his hands. He had told me he was going home but wasn't going to tell his family. It seems his brother had also lost both hands in World War II, and they didn't know it until he got off the train. I don't even know what the patient's name was but, hopefully, he's alive someplace.

Notes

[1] The V-1 program was initiated in February of 1942 for college freshmen and sophomores. Because of academic deficiencies that had become apparent in other Navy reserve training programs, the V-1 reservists were required to take at least one year of mathematics and one year of physical sciences.

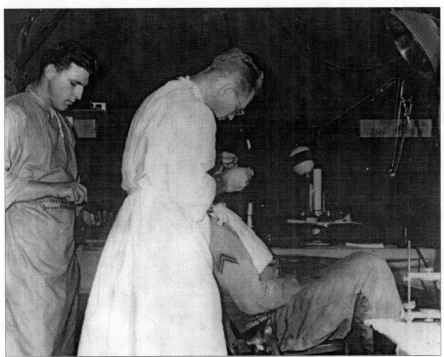

The back of a canvas-covered truck serves as a dental prosthetic unit in Korea. BUMED Archives

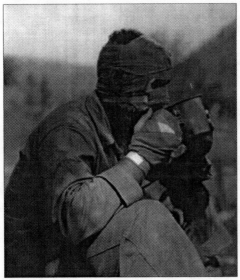

A wounded Marine sips hot coffee from a canteen cup while awaiting evacuation to a field hospital. BUMED Archives

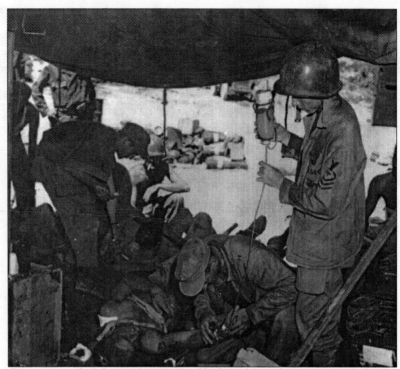

Corpsmen administer plasma at a Marine aid station somewhere near the Naktong River front, August 1950. BUMED Archives

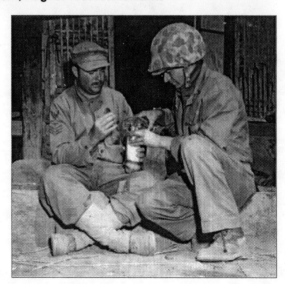

Navy corpsmen reconstitute dried blood plasma by mixing it with distilled water. BUMED Archives

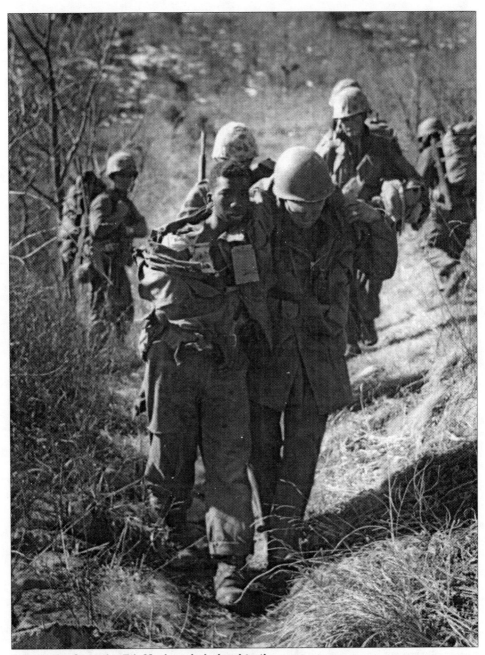

A casualty from the 7th Marines is helped to the rear. BUMED Archives

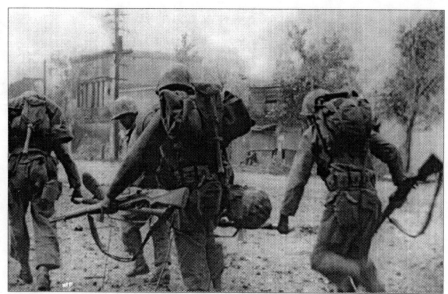

Marines carry a victim of Seoul's bitter street fighting. BUMED Archives

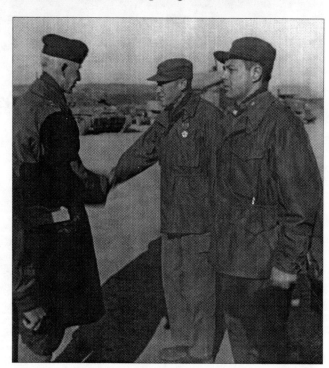

Maj. Gen. O.P. Smith, commanding officer of the 1st Marine Division, presents a gold star in lieu of a third Legion of Merit to Capt. Eugene Hering for his extraordinary service.
BUMED Archives

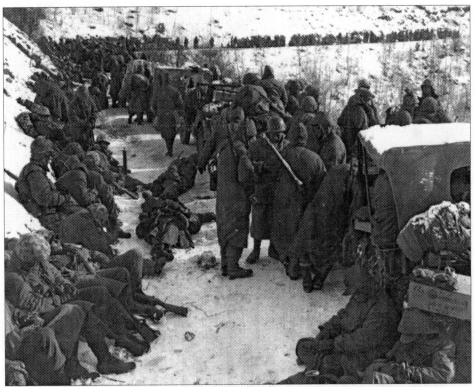

The road back from the Chosin Reservoir. BUMED Archives

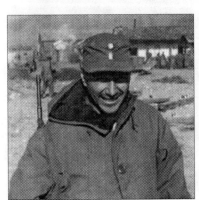

Lt.(j.g.) Morton Silver. Courtesy of
Edith Lessenden

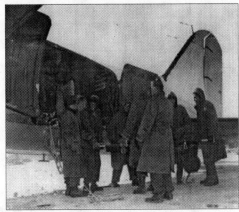

Casualties from the Chosin Reservoir
withdrawal are put aboard an R4D at
Hagaru-ri. BUMED Archives

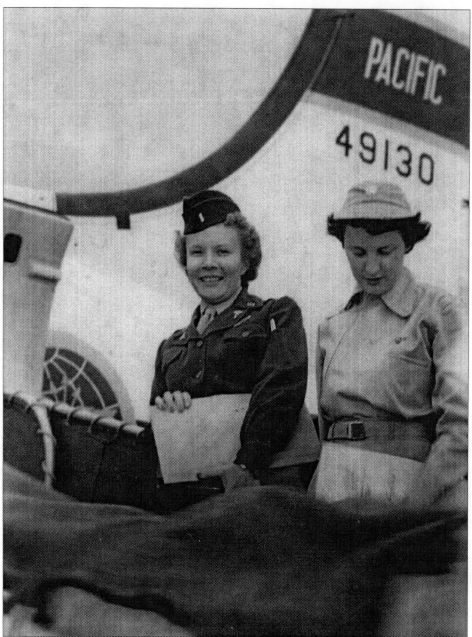

Flight nurse Lt. Bobbi Hovis (right) and an Air Force colleague supervise casualty loading aboard an evacuation aircraft. BUMED Archives

Navy nurse Lura Jane Emery cares for her Marine patient Sgt. Paul Robinson aboard USS *Repose* (AH-16). BUMED Archives

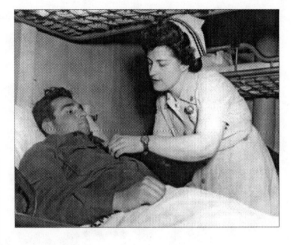

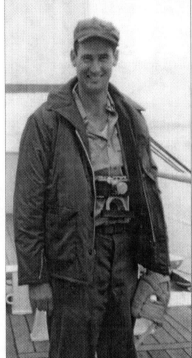

Marine pilot and Boston Red Sox star Ted Williams as a patient aboard USS *Haven*.
Nancy Crosby Collection, BUMED Archives

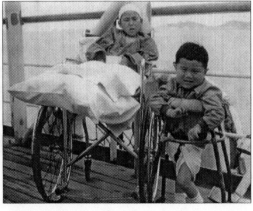

Caring for the orphan. Two young Koreans are treated aboard hospital ship *Haven*. Nancy Crosby Collection, BUMED Archives

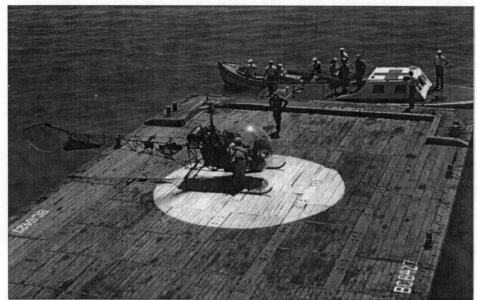

One of two barges served as USS *Haven*'s first helo decks. Nancy Crosby Collection, BUMED Archives

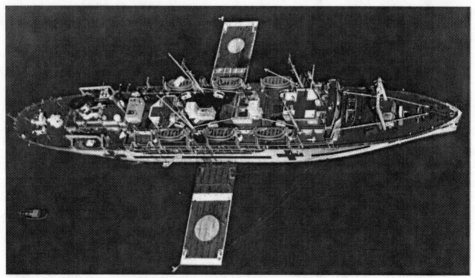

USS *Haven* lies at anchor in Inchon Harbor in the summer of 1952 looking like a giant space station with solar panels extended. A painted yellow disk on the deck of each barge marked the landing zone. BUMED Archives

5

Medevac

*G*etting casualties to medical attention in a nation with little or no infrastructure was a problem that absorbed medical planners throughout the Korean War. Many patients could not be returned to their units right away because they required at least sixty days of care. They usually went to the Naval Hospital in Yokosuka, Japan, for treatment.

Patients who needed more specialized and long-term care were evacuated to naval hospitals back in the States. Twin-engine R4Ds (C-47s) carried eighteen to twenty-four stretcher cases; four-engine C-54s had room for thirty six; and four-engine C-97s could accommodate up to one hundred casualties for medevac. Besides ensuring patients specialized treatment outside the theater of operations, air evacuation helped release the three hospital ships from extensive transport duty, allowing them to remain on station longer to serve as offshore hospitals.

Air Force flight nurse Lillian Keil flew air-evacuation missions into Hagaru during the Chosin campaign and was attached to the Air Force Combat Cargo Command's 801st Squadron. She spent most of her tour evacuating patients within Korea or to hospitals in Japan. Navy flight nurse Bobbi Hovis, flying with the joint Air Force-Navy 1453rd Medical Air Evacuation Squadron, took over from there, helping transport patients back across the Pacific.

* * *

No Fear of Flying

Lt. Cmdr. Bobbi Hovis always had two passions—nursing and aviation. At her first duty station—Naval Hospital Jacksonville, Florida—it was only natural that she join the local flying club. Before long, she had soloed in the classic yellow Piper J-3 Cub and earned her private license. After reporting to her next assignment, Naval Hospital Key West in Florida, Hovis soon became co-owner of a J-3 Cub. After the duty day was over, the young nurse and her partner would fly out to meet the submarines coming home to base. "We'd buzz the subs and they would wave and we would wave. It was great fun." In the summer of 1950, her two greatest loves would become inseparable.

On June 25th of 1950, I was on night duty at Key West Naval Hospital and, in my course of ward rounds, I went by the O.D.'s [officer of the day] office. Radio broadcasting was interrupted, and the announcer said North Korea had invaded South Korea and that we were now at war.

I had submitted my request for Navy flight nurse school sometime in '48 or '49 and received those orders in August of '50. I took a short leave, and then reported to Gunter Air Force Base, a satellite field of Maxwell Air Force Base in Montgomery, Alabama.

We had a nine-week, very intense flight nursing curriculum, and then with the war and our having to get out there to the Korean theater, that nine weeks was packed into six.

This was a combined school with Navy nurses, Air Force nurses, and one Royal Canadian Air Force nurse who went through the syllabus with us. There were our Air Force friends in the class, too, but, of course, the Navy stuck together. We were housed in the same barracks so it wasn't like I was entirely away from the Navy. Besides, we were worked to death just trying to complete the whole course in six weeks as opposed to nine. We were either studying or flying or we went to bed to get some sleep when we could.

For our student medevac flights we mostly flew in the old C-47s to places like Eglin Air Force Base where there was all-weather training in the climatic hangar. There was also cold-weather, jungle, water, and desert training. These four phases made up our survival training within various types of environments.

Air-evacing a patient is quite different from just putting a patient in an ambulance so there were things we had to know particularly unique to flight and aviation. Knowing how to properly care for head and chest injuries was a requirement because both are influenced by altitude. In those days, our flights were not in pressurized aircraft.

Sometimes there were polio patients, so we had to manage those old iron lungs. It was difficult because a 37-volt system was required in the aircraft. Not many aircraft were equipped with this system so polio flights were very special, and managing the polio patient at [high] altitude was difficult.

Then there was a concern about patients wearing heavy casts, particularly if the aircraft had to ditch over water. Actually, there would probably be very little we could do for patients in heavy plaster hip spicas—heavy shoulder casts—as far as moving them off the aircraft and into life rafts. Nevertheless, there was a lot of emphasis on ditching, survival at sea, and managing patients as far as getting them out of the aircraft and into life rafts. Our instructions were to save ourselves first so that we could care for any survivors. We learned several techniques for surviving in the water. A dead flight nurse would help no one.

Because I had a flying background before flight school, the Air Force chief nurse asked me if I would stay on their faculty to teach after graduation. Of course,

I felt quite honored, but I had worked so long and hard for my Navy flight nurse wings that I wanted to get out to the squadron and to the Korean War immediately. That's what I was trained to do. I very graciously declined the offer and told her I'd worked long and hard for this, and that I really wanted to go where the action was. She said she understood.

I immediately got my orders to the Pacific for what we called the Korean airlift. The squadron was stationed at Hickam Air Force Base in Hawaii, but we were seldom there since we island-hopped across to Japan. It was a very long flight, actually following the same routes as the glorious old Pan-American Clippers from Hickam to Johnston to Midway to Wake to Iwo Jima, and Guam. In fact, I scuba-dived much of my way across the Pacific, it seemed, because we were frequently having engine failures early on in the war. I always carried my scuba gear with me, not for ditching but to dive on the reefs of many of these islands while the aircraft was being repaired.

Medical crews would deadhead out to Japan, meaning that there were no patients aboard. As a result, we would rest as much as possible, knowing that these were going to be long, grueling flights back across the Pacific, particularly in nonpressurized aircraft.

The Navy hospital ship *Benevolence*'s sinking occurred in August of 1950, and then in September there was the C-54 crash at Kwajalein.[1] Between the two, there was a lot of tragedy as far as losing Navy nurses on their way out to the war area. On my flights back from Hawaii to Travis Air Force Base, the plane would often fly right over San Francisco Bay, and I could see that beautiful ship lying on her side with the red cross, the green stripe, and the white hull clearly visible in the sunlight. Seeing her there on the bottom and knowing that she was never going to be salvaged was heartbreaking.

My first trip across the Pacific was aboard a Berlin Airlift-vintage Air Force C-54. In fact, there was one of those old C-54s all flight crews hated to fly. Its fuselage number was 5559. We called her "Triple Nickel Nine." The pilots hated to fly her because they could never put her into perfect trim. So when the crew drew "Triple Nickel Nine," everyone threw up their hands and hoped we would make it across and back.

When we arrived at the 1453rd Medevac Squadron in Hawaii after our training, we mostly flew the old dinosaurs and junkers—C-54s and R4Ds—that had been used in the Berlin Airlift [June 1948–September 1949]. Those planes were worn out before they came to the Pacific. They still had coal dust between the cracks in the decks from all the coal that was hauled into Berlin after the war. Quite simply, this was risky equipment that perhaps we shouldn't have been flying on those long transits across the ocean. But there was little choice. I rarely completed a mission on four engines.

Later the Air Force received new C-97 Boeing Stratocruisers, which were pure luxury. They had a very high patient capacity compared to what we were used to. Because stretchers were stacked five high, it was difficult to administer nursing care to the patients on the top stretchers.

Our medical kits were quite large and they weighed about sixty pounds. We would drag along the medical kit and then stand on it to reach those top-level patients. We always tried to place patients requiring the least nursing care at that level, or the tallest of us would take care of them. Often, a tall corpsman would be assigned those patients.

It was very grueling as far as rest was concerned. In fact, there was very little rest at all. It was a twenty-four-hour, round-the-clock flight operation. As it turned out, the winter of 1950 was the worst on record in both Japan and Korea. That was in December of 1950, and we lost a lot of Marines who fought at the infamous battlefield of the Chosin Reservoir. There were Army men lost as well, but I seem to remember only Marine patients. They were not well prepared for such a severe winter and fighting such an overwhelming battle with the North Koreans and Chinese. There were entire planeloads of patients without another type of wound except frostbite of the hands and feet.

In order to bring those frostbitten patients back in the best possible state, and in an attempt to save those fingers, toes, feet, and hands, we had to keep the cabin very cool—probably in the low forties, as I recall—so the medical crews were unbearably cold.[2]

Medical flight crews weren't really adequately dressed. We flight nurses wore a Navy leather flight jacket over the top of our aviation uniform green jacket and that was it. To keep those cabins as cool as we did, we would rotate—"we" meaning the medical crews. Some stayed with the patients while others went up to the flight deck to warm up. Needless to say, there was a high rate of pneumonia, severe colds, and URIs [upper respiratory infections] throughout the medical crew members, particularly those on the frostbite flights.

After the C-97s came on line, there were enough litters for about a hundred patients, as I recall. And these frostbite patients often had a lot of pain, as well as early gangrene. We treated their pain and tried to keep them as comfortable as possible, using morphine and Demerol for pain control. There wasn't much else we could do for them. If their dressings were weeping, which many of them were, dressings were changed as necessary. We could only try to keep them comfortable and warm. It seemed as though we used tons of blankets in that very cool cabin. Many of these Marines went to the Amputation Center at Oakland Naval Hospital in California.

On a typical flight, we deadheaded from Hickam and island-hopped to Japan, landing at Haneda Air Force Base in Tokyo, the former Japanese air base the U.

S. took over during the occupation. A flight to Japan might take fifteen to twenty hours because of fuel stops at several islands. Most of us would lie down on litters and try to get some rest on the way out.

Once we landed at Haneda, we fell into bed and got up the next morning to make the trip to Yokosuka Naval Station, some distance from Tokyo. The Yokosuka shipyard was where the naval hospital was located. We then got a list of our air-evac patients. There was a chief nurse stationed at Haneda, and she coordinated with the naval hospital as to which patients would be assigned to this particular aircraft that just arrived.

Our list of patients was screened at Yokosuka. This meant visiting every patient and reviewing his medical history with the ward medical officer—frostbite, gunshot wound, whatever. The doctor then briefed us on specific things to watch for in flight because we nurses and corpsmen were the only medical personnel aboard.

About 0850 in the morning we introduced ourselves to the patients. Usually our flight was scheduled for a 1600 takeoff. When the briefings were finished, we returned to quarters at Haneda and waited until it was time for patient loading.

At the flight line, lines of ambulances from Naval Hospital Yokosuka awaited us. We then boarded the plane. Most of us had already planned in our minds which spot in the aircraft a particular patient would be assigned. In the C-97s, for example, I wanted those patients requiring more nursing care to be on the second or third tier because that was the easiest level to work from. Lower down or on the deck, your back would break, leaning over to care for a patient. The most critical and those requiring the most nursing care were always placed at a level where it was easier to take care of them. After all were strapped in, we briefed them for takeoff, and soon were taxiing out, cleared for takeoff, and then heading back across the Pacific.

Guam was a staging area, and often those patients in the worst condition would be off-loaded at Guam and taken to Guam Naval Hospital at Naval Air Station Agaña, where they were bathed, fed, and their dressings changed.

There was a staging area on Midway Island. The patients weren't off-loaded. Instead, the "Gray Ladies" and other volunteers on the island came to the aircraft while the flight crews went to a lounge or some other area for a few hours rest or a meal. The volunteers then helped change dressings and feed the patients.

The thought of water ditching was always with us, especially because of patients in heavy body casts. On one flight from Korea to Hawaii an engine failed. Then about a hundred miles out of Hickam, we lost a second engine. And here we were with a fully loaded aircraft! Needless to say, there was a glaring possibility of losing a third engine. Hickam dispatched two air-sea rescue aircraft which took up station, one on our port and the other on our starboard wing. Well, it was very reassuring to see those aircraft off each of our wings, but if we had to ditch, all they could do would be to radio our location and initiate rescue operations. The Douglas aircraft were really old workhorses. Altitude could be maintained on two engines. But if a third engine were lost, we were in big trouble.

There was a great sigh of relief when our crew received a direct emergency final approach clearance from the tower. There were all types of rescue equipment—ambulances, cranes, foam-trucks, and fire engines—following us down the runway. When the aircraft rolled to a stop and the engines—all two of them—were shut down, we knew our guardian angels were on duty that day. And no, we were not flying "Triple Nickel Nine."

One of my C-97 flights would prove to be quite unnerving. We were outbound from Hickam with twenty or so nurses and techs deadheading to Haneda. Cabin lights were dim, flight boots and shoes were lined up neatly on the deck, as most of us were resting on the litters. Even though mostly asleep, I was constantly aware of engine sounds. I think all people who fly airplanes—the pilots—in the backs of our minds we are constantly tuned to a proper synchronized engine sound, and when it's not there, or absent altogether, we suddenly become aware of it. Suddenly, there was total silence aboard this aircraft. I was instantly awake as the C-97 began a precipitous imitation of a falling brick. That aircraft had the glide ratio of a rock. Shoes and boots began bouncing off the overhead in wild disarray. Everyone in a litter slammed upward, crashing into the litter directly above. As the aircraft headed directly for the Pacific, one engine finally caught and restarted, followed quickly by the other three. Anyone care to guess the cause? The crew forgot to switch fuel tanks. Fortunately for us, a midair engine start was achieved. There were a number of bumps and bruises and bloody noses. By the time we got forty or so boots and shoes sorted out, we were so wired that additional sleep was impossible.

Later, when I was assigned to the Navy's VR-2 squadron, the aircraft I really liked was the Martin Mars, the huge JRM flying boats operating between John Rogers Naval Air Station, adjacent to Hickam Air Force Base in Hawaii, and Alameda Naval Air Station in California. A Mars could carry three times as many ambulatory patients as any other existing aircraft. Flight time west to east was about twelve to fourteen hours at about 170 miles an hour. Because the patients were ambulatory, nursing duties were minimal aboard these flights, that is, administering medications and inspections, some dressing changes, and assisting patients using crutches.

The Mars was special and unique. Its wingspan was 200 feet and the fuselage was 120 feet long. The wing root, where it joined the fuselage, was so large that I could stand fully erect and walk out into the interior of the wing. All four engines could be accessed and serviced from within the wing structure. I flew aboard the *Caroline Mars*. There were four others plus the prototype. One of the Mars aircraft once carried an entire carrier air group, which was about 301, plus 7, from

Alameda, California, to San Diego. The Mars had a 100 percent safety record. In fifteen years of flying, it logged eighty-seven thousand hours.

Notes

[1]On 20 August 1950, the four-engine C-54, en route to Japan, crashed on take off and sank in 7,200 feet of water off Kwajalein in the Marshall Islands. All twenty-six Navy personnel aboard perished, including eleven Navy nurses recently recalled to active duty and slated for assignments at Naval Hospital Yokosuka. These Navy nurses were Ensign Eleanor C. Beste, Ensign Marie M. Boatman, Lt.(j.g.) Jeanne E. Clarke, Lt.(j.g.) Jane L. Eldridge, Ensign Constance R. Esposito, Lt.(j.g.) Alice S. Giroux, Lt.(j.g.) Calla V. Goodwin, Lt.(j.g.) Constance A. Heege, Lt.(j.g.) Margaret G. Kennedy, Ensign Mary E. Liljegreen, and Ensign Edna J. Rundell.

[2]It was felt at the time that rewarming frostbitten tissue too rapidly might result in further injury.

6

The *Haven* Sisters

*W*hen the United Nations responded to the Korean crisis with troops in the first days of July 1950, military medical assets in that theater of war did not exist. The vast Pacific network of fleet, mobile, and base hospitals the Navy had painstakingly knit together during World War II unraveled with victory. But as the Korean fighting grew intense and the closest naval hospital was in Japan, another option was required—hospital ships.

By 1945, the Navy hospital ship fleet had grown from but two vessels at the time of Pearl Harbor to fifteen white hulls. Now, except for one, USS Consolation *(AH-15), all these mercy ships had been sold, scrapped, or mothballed. Even as* Consolation *arrived at besieged Pusan in July 1950, USS* Benevolence *(AH-13) was being readied for action. But unlucky hull 13 never arrived. On 25 August 1950, the ship was returning from a shakedown cruise in San Francisco Bay prior to her upcoming departure for Korea. About four miles from the Golden Gate, an outward bound freighter, SS* Mary Luckenbach, *suddenly emerged from the fog. Her bow struck the hospital ship's port side, sliced through her thin steel plates, slid down her side, and sheared the hull again amidships.* Benevolence *took an immediate list, slowly turned on her beam ends, and sank in less than half an hour. Of the 518 aboard, 23 perished. One of the survivors, nurse Ensign Dorothy Venverloh, recounts the incident.*

* * *

Unlucky AH-13

I was at Oak Knoll [Naval Hospital, Oakland, California] on a surgical ward when we heard they were having troubles in Korea. My orders were dated the 25th of July 1950, and I and another nurse had to report to Mare Island Naval Shipyard [Vallejo, California] because that's where the *Benevolence* was in mothballs. Our assignment was with the Reserve Fleet for temporary duty. We reported in and then lived in Quonset huts on the base because the Mare Island hospital was officially closed two weeks before.

One of the hospital chiefs from the Naval Hospital in Houston was on duty there aboard the hospital ship so he showed us all around—above deck, below deck, the elevators, and then when we got down below where the hospital units were, he said, "This ship is not as seaworthy as some of the other ships." I always kept what he said in the back of my mind.

The ship looked like it had been taken care of pretty well. Just as the wool blankets were preserved with camphor (mothballs), the remainder of the ship had been protected by spraying it with layers to protect it and to "cocoon" it when it was placed in the "Mothball" fleet.

I was very excited about being assigned to a hospital ship. That was one of the things one always thought about. This was choice duty for a nurse. I had come into the Navy in '47 and, of course, many of the experienced personnel had been released to inactive duty.

We were to go aboard earlier but couldn't because this was going to be the first ship that sailed with a Navy crew and a merchant marine crew. The merchant mariners had gotten there first, staked out their territory, and took over the staterooms. So the [officers] had to find a different place for them and get them moved out. We weren't too sure just how this was all going to work out. It was said the [crewmen] were very resentful because when they had moved aboard, no one had told them anything. Anyway, we finally got moved aboard.

Our staterooms were about the size of the back hall upstairs at home. We had bunk beds. I slept in the upper—a metal cabinet. We each had a combination desk–chest of drawers with a built-in safe. Our stateroom had a sink against the one bulkhead and the medicine chest on the other wall. The movements of more than one person in the room had to be timed.

The first day we were to go out on a shakedown cruise. Afterward, the plan was to return to Mare Island and load up with supplies. Then we were going to Korea to relieve the *Consolation*. We would have stayed on the ship that night before sailing for Korea the next day.

On Friday, we were nosed out of the berth by two tugs and then proceeded on our way. We left Mare Island at 0800 and throughout the morning we frequently were on deck just to see what was to be seen. Prior to this, we hadn't yet had "abandon ship" or lifeboat drills. We didn't have them until after we moved aboard. On that shakedown cruise down the bay, we went to the officers' mess, where the captain read the orders taking the ship from the Reserve fleet and putting it back on active duty. The chief nurse told us she had our lifeboat assignments and would give them to us the next day.

We passed Treasure Island around 1100 and then went under the San Francisco-Oakland Bay Bridge into San Francisco Bay. The ship's engines and equipment were being tested. The ship circled, turned around, speeded up, slowed down, etc., for about two hours. Then about 1400 we sailed back under the Bay Bridge. Slightly off Treasure Island they tested the anchors, etc. While all this testing was being done by the sailors and the civil service crew, who were to take over when the ship returned to Mare Island, the plumbers, pipefitters, carpenters, and painters were attempting to finish up their work so the ship would be ready to turn over to the Military Sea Transport Service [MSTS] when we returned to Mare Island. There were several civil service and port observers along to check on various equipment, to check the radar, to calibrate the compass, etc.

We then headed toward the Golden Gate Bridge. Although it was about 1500, the fog, which enshrouds the Golden Gate Bridge and lies outside the Golden Gate, was already so dense when we went under the bridge, the lower part of the bridge could scarcely be seen until we were quite near to it.

When we got out beyond the bridge, we were on deck most of the time. We stayed out so much because the motion of the ship could be felt more when we were indoors and one of the girls was starting to complain of nausea.

On the trials outside the Golden Gate Bridge the ship had to make figures of 8 and the boilers had to be run at 40, 60, and 80 percent of full capacity. About 1645, one of the MSTS boys came down from the bridge of the ship and said, "Maybe we'll get back to Mare Island in time for some liberty; we're going to turn around soon." The fog had gotten progressively thicker, and we had hung over the rail discussing how easy it would be to miss seeing anyone who might be in the water. Little did we know!

Anyway, we were getting ready to go to dinner at 1700 hours. Our mess was on the next deck down. Just about then I heard this long whistle blast and felt a severe jarring, like a hard earthquake tremor. I stepped to the porthole but couldn't see anything, so, being a woman and nosy, I grabbed my coat and started down the passageway to the deck to see what happened. Two of the other girls came dashing along, too. We got partially out to the boat deck when we were hit again. We got out the door, and when we felt how much the ship was listing, we said one to another, "Whatever's happened, it isn't good. Let's close this outside [watertight] door."

We started back to our quarters and that was when we heard, "Prepare to abandon ship. Get your life jackets. Report to the starboard side. Close all watertight doors." The dishes in the dining room [wardroom] were all clanking and clattering and breaking. Some of the trunks that had not been placed in the trunk room slid back and forth in the passageway.

We did not know very much about what was going on. We knew the ship was listing and not stabilized. We were all so busy getting out of our quarters. There was someone who didn't take her life jacket, and she wanted somebody to bring her one. Prior to this, most of the life jackets had been gathered and placed on another deck. They were to be sent out to be cleaned that very day so some people didn't have them in their rooms. But we had ours. We had thrown them on top of the metal cabinet in our stateroom.

Then they told us to be sure to put our life jackets on. When we had our indoctrination course, nothing much was said about putting on life jackets. You know, you put this thing on and then you wrap this long tape around you and tie the knot in it. Well, we had never been told that you were supposed to secure some of the straps between the legs. And, of course, we were wearing full skirts—uniforms. So most of us just tied the strap around our waist. Well, that resulted in difficulty later on when we were in the water because the life jackets had a tendency to ride upward and float over your head. We were never taught how to wear the life jackets. Maybe they assumed we should know by common sense. The men knew what to do with them but we didn't.

By the time we got back to try to get to the boat deck, the ship had already listed so much one of the men held onto the side of the doorway and stretched his hand in to us, and by joining hands we were assisted up to the passageway. By clinging to the railing along the passageway we got out to the outer decks.

The men were feverishly trying to get the lifeboats down but this job proved futile, as the ship listed more and more. Some of the men joined hands and helped us up to the railing and told us to climb through. By this time the rafts had been dumped, but had not been attached by rope to the side of the ship as they apparently should have been, so they had floated quite a distance out empty. Many of the crew, corpsmen, doctors, etc., went off the ship and swam out to the rafts and climbed into them. But because they had no oars, they were unable to get back to the ship.

Someone came out and told us to relax, saying that "even if the ship settles, we are only in forty-eight feet of water and the ship is seventy-two feet wide."

So we proceeded to sit on the top rail with our feet braced on the middle rail just like in the bleachers, thinking, "This won't be so bad. We'll just wait until someone picks us up—kind of like waiting for a streetcar."

The ship kept rolling over and soon we heard steam hissing. We knew the boilers had been secured before the men left, but when we heard the hissing and all, the captain told us to move down on the ship away from the area of the engine room.

The ship by this time was practically on its side. The men were still trying to get the lifeboats down but whatever held them could not be released with the ship over so far. By this time the waves were lapping up over the hull.

In the meantime, Capt. [Cecil] Riggs, the medical CO, who was still aboard, had some of the men go around and get wooden planks to put into the water. Planks and coils of rope and round life preservers were available for "man overboard" drills. The idea was that we needed something to hang on to. While we were on deck, he ran the rope through the belt loops on the back of our coats. In fact, we were wearing everything—full skirted uniforms, hats, sweaters, coats, and purses. After all, we were going somewhere.

They finally told us to get off the ship, and we had to navigate our way down the side. We all got a hand on the wood and stepped off the bilge keel into the water. Those of us who were close to the ship braced our feet against the bottom of the ship to push away. With that a huge wave came along, picked us up, and carried us a good distance away.

The boards in the water were pretty wide—about eighteen inches or so—and quite thick. I had a death grip on the board I was holding on to. When the men on the ocean-going tug finally pulled me out, I couldn't bend my left hand for a good day. I was holding on to my roommate Rosemary with my other hand because her arms weren't long enough to reach the board. She was holding on to me and I was holding on to the board. Some of the merchant seamen were holding on to the opposite side of our board.

As we stepped off into the water, the Chief Nurse, [Lt.] Nell Harrington said, "Don't people abandoning ship always sing? Let's sing." So she started "Merrily We Roll Along." The reaction of most of us to singing at a time like that was not too dramatic. We all felt we should save our breath and our strength, and there was less danger of getting saltwater in our mouths if we kept them closed.

Nell said to the girl next to her, Eileen Dyer, "Why don't you sing with us?"

And Eileen said, "I'm too busy praying." So we all were quiet except that all the Catholic nurses were praying more or less audibly.

Josephine McCarthy would call to me every once in a while, "Are you all right Dorothy?" And as time went by, and our life jackets worked up around our ears, the neck string was up under my nose. My hat was down over my eyes. By raising my eyebrows to raise my hat, I could see just barely over the edge of the life jacket. I was holding on for dear life, paddling my feet and with the blue dye of the life jackets falling onto our faces and necks.

As I was in this fine array, Rosemary looked over at me and said, "Dorothy, are you comfortable?"

I remember one of the men saying, "Well, that's one way to consider it."

Every once in a while we'd hear the mournful clang of a buoy bell. I never did see the buoy. Once we saw just a ghostlike outline of a fishing boat. It apparently didn't see or hear us, although we shouted and waved a free hand.

We were tiring rapidly. Even the men who had been doggedly cheerful expressed the thought that if we weren't picked up soon, we couldn't last the night. The water was getting colder, it seemed. I think we later learned that it was around fifty degrees. It was harder for us to kick our legs. We also heard that had we been in that water just ten minutes more, they would have pulled our bodies out. It was also rough. First we'd be down in a trough, and then we'd be way up, and then down. It was so foggy and we were so intent on holding on that we didn't see the ship go under.

After a while we saw the captain's gig come up and one of the sailors aboard said, "I can't take you aboard, but I'll tell them where you are." Apparently he had a tough time keeping the engine running.

About that time an Army Engineer tug appeared and the crew fired a Very [flare] pistol over us and told us to catch the line. They shot several lines to us but we missed them. Finally they shot one directly across Rosemary, me, Wilma Ledbetter , and the men on the other side of the board raft, and another line across the other end of the raft. We hung on and they pulled us to the tug. Wilma kept fighting the line with which they were trying to pull us in. Every time she would shout, her head would dip into the water. Finally someone from the tug jumped in to hold her up, but she wouldn't cooperate. We tried to tell the men we were tied together. They tried to pull us aboard, but with the sloshing of the waves we would slide right out of their grasp. And we didn't have the strength to cling to their hands. One of the men from the tug jumped in the water and cut the rope between each of us so they were able to pull us individually up over the side of the tug. I would have been the last person pulled aboard except that Wilma didn't let them come near her. We were trying to do that, but Wilma kept pushing them away saying they were going to drown her. She was very panicky. So they turned their attention to me instead. When the waves washed me up high, two men, who were hanging over the railing, each grabbed one of my arms and pulled me up over the side.

Wilma, then, ended up being last. She continued to fight them as they tried to pull her out of the water and, by the time they finally got her aboard, her color was terrible, kind of a pinkish-blue, and she wasn't responding. She died aboard that tugboat, probably from hypothermia.

They helped me on deck and stood me on my feet and said, "Are you OK?" And I thought I was and started to walk to the back of the tug. I got about ten or twelve feet and remember stumbling into a stack of wet life jackets. One of the boys came along and helped me down into the engine room of the tug. It was jammed like sardines. Two of the nurses were down there. They helped me take off my coat and sweater. The men moved to let me lean against the engine to try to warm up. Most of the men had stripped to their trunks trying to get warm and dry their clothes. In trying to find out the time, I discovered my watch was still running. It was 7:10 P.M.

Soon thereafter, they brought the pilot down on some boards. We later learned that he had been thrown back against the wheel on the bridge and had seriously injured his back when the collision occurred. I don't think he survived.[1]

They took as many people as they could aboard the tug and returned to the pier in San Francisco. At first, not all the nurses were accounted for. [Ensign] Helen Wallis was with a merchant seaman who had survived several shipwrecks in the past. The ship that hit us pulled out survivors who were floating in its path. Helen was one of those and was brought to our ward at Oak Knoll some time later.

We were taken to Oak Knoll [Naval Hospital] on buses where we were admitted. We stayed for several days and were put to work on the wards until all our paperwork was reconstructed. We lost all of that except for our pay records, which weren't aboard.

Some time later we had to go back to Mare Island for a closed meeting of the people who had been aboard the ship. We weren't supposed to talk to anybody about what was discussed. They told each of us that if there was someone we wanted to praise or condemn for their actions, that was the time to do it.

The next day they took us to Treasure Island to get some uniforms. We had lost everything but what we were wearing. I have the purse I had with me right here, and it's stiff and still has the salt on it.

What's peculiar about all this is that no one ever talked to me about the sinking. The first time anybody really mentioned the event was at my separation interview. And that was about 1970.

For a long time the memories of that day kept bugging me. Why couldn't we have done more to keep Wilma with us? Some of the girls were talking to her. Some of them were praying with her. I don't really know what more we could have done to save her.

There's also another memory. When I was sinking through my life jacket and Rosemary reached over and pulled the tie down farther, I had an out-of-body experience. When I looked downward, I could see the side of the ship with a few ant-sized bodies moving and many ant-sized bodies in the water moving away from the ship. When I was looking upward, I heard harp-like music and saw a translucent stairway going up to the heavens. I didn't see anybody up there. I had ascended almost to the top of the stairs, and a voice asked me if I was all right. And that brought me back, back to being in the water with Rosemary. I've often wondered what I would have found at the top of those stairs.

On 11 January 1951, a U.S. Coast Guard board of inquiry released its findings. Because of dense fog, Benevolence *was using her radar. However, the radar equipment on* Mary Luckenbach *was malfunctioning and had been shut down. Even though both vessels were sounding regulation fog signals, they were proceeding at excessive speeds. At the moment of impact, the hospital ship was making fifteen knots, the freighter, about twelve knots. A total of twenty-five minutes had elapsed from the time of collision until the vessel sank. The first list to port was followed by a further listing and settling by the head, bringing the main deck to sea level within five minutes. The* Benevolence *then remained somewhat stationary at about a forty-five-degree list and slowly capsized on her port side.*

Coast Guard inspectors were unable to determine the damage below the waterline, but they reported in detail the fatal damage they could see: "A hole extending upwards, five to ten feet high, from three to five feet above the water line and in length from frame 50 aft to about frame 72 or 77, a distance of about fifty feet, with one or two strakes of shell plating ripped out. This resulted almost immediately in flooding compartments between frames 13 and 32, 32 and 56, 56 and 82, and possibly aft of frame 82."[2]

Although there was enough blame to go around, the Coast Guard report cited the Navy for failure to train the crew or to conduct any fire, collision, and abandon-ship drills before proceeding to the open sea. Because the commanding officer misjudged the seriousness of the collision, he failed to order "abandon ship" immediately, which resulted in delayed efforts to launch lifeboats. As a result, the serious list precluded the launching of any of the hospital ship's twelve lifeboats; only the after starboard motor whaleboat was released.

The Coast Guard also found that an SOS sent immediately after the collision was futile as the antenna had been previously disconnected.

Of nine Navy personnel assigned to security patrol, eight were either eating or on the chow line at the time of the collision. Because of the absence of these men from their stations, they were unable to execute the commanding officer's order to close the watertight doors.

The following morning, the white-hulled hospital ship rested on her side in seventy feet of water, her red crosses plainly visible. The San Francisco Daily News *described the melancholy scene. "Now . . . only the tangled lifeboats were above the water's surface—these and the crosses, which glared redly through the greenish water in the trough of each swell."[3]*

* * *

Out of Mothballs

The day following the Benevolence *tragedy, Chief of Naval Operations Adm. Forrest Sherman ordered the reactivation of USS* Haven *(AH-12) to replace her lost sister. The last action* Haven *had seen after her debut in World War II was participation in "Operation Cross Roads," the nuclear tests at the Bikini atoll in 1946. Also helping to take up the slack was USS* Repose *(AH-16), which soon joined* Haven *and* Consolation *in Korea.[4]*

The three Haven-class hospital ships, which were reactivated for the Korean crisis, had been converted during World War II from C-4 freighter hulls. They were built by Sun Shipbuilding and Dry Dock Company of Chester, Pennsylvania, and taken over by the Navy while still under construction. Consolation, Haven, *and* Repose *were complete, state-of-the art afloat hospitals in every respect. With operating rooms, clinics, laboratories, treatment rooms, and wards, and staffed by specialists, these mercy ships were comparable or superior to most modern, contemporary hospitals ashore. They were equipped to provide definitive surgical and medical care.*

The Haven *sisters were almost identical. Each 520-foot-long hull had a beam of seventy-two feet and displaced 11,400 tons. With its single screw nine thousand-shaft horsepower, geared turbine drive, each ship had a top speed of eighteen knots. Each ship had eight decks, three below the water line. All machinery spaces were located aft, leaving the entire forward portion of the vessels available for hospital spaces. This arrangement allowed the hospital to be one unit, not built around the uptake spaces and machinery trunks, as in conventional ships. All treatment rooms and wards could be accessed by wide, continuous corridors.*

The surgical suite, clinics, and treatment rooms were in the center of the ship where movement from pitch and roll was minimized. The surgical suite included two major operating rooms, a fracture operating room, an anesthesia room, surgical supply room, clinical laboratory, and dispensary.

In the central surgical supply room and its adjacent spaces, cleaning, processing, and sterilizing surgical equipment was stored for all operating rooms and wards. Passageways in the surgical suite were designed to permit use of the supply room, dispensary, and laboratory by wards and clinics in other parts of the ship when operations were being performed.

The eye, ear, nose, and throat department, patterned after successful shore installations, was equipped with its own operating room. If necessary, this area could be used as a general operating room, three treatment rooms, one refraction room, or one examination room.

Each vessel had an optical repair unit to provide and repair eyeglasses. The dental clinic had its own fully equipped laboratory and x-ray and darkroom facilities. The radiology department included a record and appointment office, examination room, and x-ray machines. All spaces were lead-lined to prevent radiation leakage. Other hospital facilities included a dermatology clinic, a physiotherapy department, and additional laboratories.

The hospital complement for each ship allowed for twenty-five physicians, three dentists, thirty nurses, four Medical Service Corps officers, and two hundred hospital corpsmen. The staff also included dental, laboratory, and operating technicians and opticians.

Haven-*class hospital ships were the first Navy vessels to be air conditioned throughout the living and hospital spaces. Because the crew and medical staff quarters, surgical suite, treatment rooms, and most medical offices were located below the waterline, the entire upper deck was available for wards and recreational spaces.*

The ships' messing arrangements were also state of the art. Patients' meals arrived from the galley by food elevators. Diet pantries in the wards had vacuum food containers, electric steam tables, and heated cabinets for keeping food hot.

Each vessel had seventy-eight beds in locked wards, sixty-eight beds in isolation wards, seventy-eight marine heads (toilets), eighty sinks, and forty-one showers in its hospital spaces. These ships could accommodate 780 patients. Compared to earlier times, Haven-class patients were truly pampered. Most hospital bunks were eventually furnished with headphones, and the patient had a choice of four radio programs. Those patients too incapacitated to write could use a recorder to send his "voice letter" back home. There were also regular movies and the occasional USO show.

By international convention and agreement at Geneva, hospital ships were clearly marked. The World War II scheme had a green horizontal band running fore and aft on either side, one red cross amidships, and other red crosses painted on stacks and decks. The Korean War paint job retained the green band and other markings, but the Haven-class hulls now sported three red crosses port and starboard.

These updated vessels were not employed as "ambulance ships," as were their World War II predecessors. Those ships' main function had been to stabilize and then transport casualties to more definitive care at base and mobile hospitals in the Pacific or Stateside. Although ferrying patients back to Naval Hospital Yokosuka in Japan became routine for the Haven *sisters, surgery and other treatment aboard the hospital ships returned many a Marine, soldier, and sailor to his units at the front.*

In the early stages of the Korean War, patients arrived aboard the hospital ships from the battlefield via assorted landing craft or any other small vessel that could be pressed into use. At Pusan, where Consolation *lay pierside as a station hospital, ambulances and trucks transported the wounded to the dock. While the Inchon operation was under way,* Consolation *remained offshore not only to be out of artillery range, but also because Inchon's notorious tidal range prevented her from getting any closer.*

As during World War II, small boats and landing craft ferried casualties from Inchon's invasion beaches. Some of these small craft were ship equipment. Each Haven-class vessel carried two LCPLs (Landing Craft Personnel Large), two thirty-six-foot motor launches, and two twenty-six-foot motor whaleboats for use as ambulance boats.

The technique for bringing patients aboard became highly refined. As small boats arrived alongside, a jib crane fitted with an electric winch dropped its wire slings and quickly hoisted litter- or chair-borne patients aboard. Each ship had several such jib cranes for use as litter hoists. Davits, one port and one starboard, were each capable of hoisting aboard an LCVP (Landing Craft Vehicle and Personnel) or other boats loaded with patients. Special slings and pallets permitted the use of cargo booms for hoisting litters in the event other methods could not be employed. The highline method was used to transfer patients from other vessels to the hospital ship at sea.

Open deck areas in the vicinity of the jib cranes, davits, and later, helicopter landing platforms facilitated rapid movement of patients to the ship's interior. Wide, continuous passageways further speeded stretcher movement. Gently sloping ladders and two elevators on each vessel enabled the rapid transport of patients. Three stretchers could be handled in each elevator at one time by use of a special dolly which permitted the stacking of stretchers.

Once patients were safely aboard, their prognoses relied upon highly trained physicians, nurses, and hospital corpsmen entrusted with their care. One such caregiver was Eleanor Harrington. It was "Nell" Harrington, senior nurse of the ill-fated Benevolence, *who had tried to cheer her fellow nurses in the water while awaiting rescue. Of those survivors, only she got another chance to serve aboard a hospital ship. That vessel was* Haven. *Two days after the loss of* Benevolence, Haven *was hurriedly removed from mothballs in San Diego, towed to the Long Beach Naval Shipyard, and recommissioned. In a manuscript prepared for publication in the* American Journal of Nursing, *Harrington described the duty that almost every Navy nurse yearned for.*

* * *

"Man Your Stations"

The familiar fog hanging over the Bay Area shrouded San Francisco in a gray mist. Aboard the U.S. hospital ship *Haven*, the order came clearly over the ship's intercommunication system, "Go to your stations, all the special sea detail." Shortly afterward, the ship backed away from the pier and once again sailed under the Golden Gate Bridge to commence her second tour of duty in the Far East. She carried a staff of 30 nurses. Some were reserves recently recalled to active duty; sailing on a hospital ship was a new experience for most of them. Although they all knew their destination, no one at that particular time spoke of it. They were busy getting acclimated to their new surroundings. Before long they were used to shipboard living, acquainted with their shipmates, and quite familiar with many of the nautical terms.

The USS *Haven* is a floating hospital that can accommodate 795 patients. She can be moved to any port where her facilities are needed. Besides the nursing staff, she carries a staff of 25 doctors, 3 Medical Service Corps officers, 194 hospital corpsmen, 3 dental officers, and 6 dental corpsmen in addition to the line crew, whose teamwork is always at our beck and call.

The day began with the announcement to the crew over the "squawk box," "Reveille, Reveille, all hands heave out and trice up. The smoking lamp is lighted in all authorized spaces." After a hearty breakfast, each corpsman proceeded to his particular job assignment—some to the wards, others to the various clinics.

The 18 wards aboard the ship vary in size and will take from 26 to 58 patients. The double-decker bunks have comfortable mattresses. The orthopedic wards are equipped with fracture beds, which are able to care for any necessary traction. All lower bunks throughout the ship have regular standard hospital frames, and can be adjusted to the needs and comfort of the patient. Small trays fastened to the bunks serve as bedside trays to care for the patient's personal wants. The bunks are equipped with a bedside lamp, as well as ear phones, which enables the patient to hear the transcribed programs from the Armed Forces Radio Service and the religious services from the improvised chapel. Most of the wards have their own diet kitchen equipped with electric food-warming tables. This ensures the serving of piping hot food. Every convenience is provided for the welfare and comfort of the patient. Also included in the hospital spaces are three large operating rooms, pathology laboratory, specially manned x-ray department, and physiotherapy. An EENT (eye, ear, nose, and throat) clinic is equipped with its own operating room and optical laboratory. A complete dental clinic and the latest in electrocardiographic and encephalographic machines complete a modern general hospital.

At last we reached Pusan, our home port for several months. Here our primary responsibilities were to provide nursing care for the troops of the United Nations Forces. Our sister ship, the *Consolation*, was waiting for us to relieve her. As we approached her, a military band on her flight deck welcomed us with, "If I Knew You Were Coming, I'd 'a' Baked a Cake." This became our theme song in Korea.

At first view, Pusan was a conglomeration of rectangular huts clustered by the thousands along dirty paths. Koreans squatted impassively in the doorways of their dimly-lighted huts. This was the place of refuge for thousands of Koreans who had been left homeless by the war.

During the time the ship was tied to the pier, patients were received by boat, hospital train, and ambulance. A doctor, nurse, and four corpsmen were assigned to each ward. The nurses worked eight-hour watches, on rotation, being on duty every fourth day. This meant that they must be available when a new group of patients arrived. When many casualties were to be admitted, every one reported back to her duty station. We were forewarned of the arrival of patients by the announcement, "Litter and embarkation teams, man your stations."

The embarkation officer, a physician, screened the arriving stretcher cases. He evaluated the condition of the patient as to type of wounds, injuries, or disease, and then determined to which service, ward, and bunk (upper or lower) he was to be assigned. Ambulatory patients were admitted through the record office.

As soon as a patient arrived on the ward, the nurse and a corpsman greeted him. The next immediate task was to clean him up. Sometimes this was quite a task, too, especially if the patient had been in his bunker when he was hit. After he had been scrubbed from head to toe, he was comfortably tucked between white sheets under the protective care and observation of an ever-attentive nurse who symbolized "home" to many. The anguished expression on his countenance disappeared to be replaced by a pathetic, appreciative little smile.

The wounded were usually kept aboard the ship approximately three weeks, depending on the seriousness of their injuries. Then they were transported by plane to hospitals in Japan and, shortly afterward, they were air-evacuated to the states. Navy and Marine patients were sent to the U.S. Naval Hospital in Oakland, California, and then transferred to the military hospital nearest their home. However, many patients could be returned to their own units directly from the hospital ship.

Since many of our patients were Koreans, we had need to comprehend and to try to interpret customs and language strange to all of us. Two names, Lee and Kim, appeared most often on our records.

One Lee, like all patients on admission, received a short haircut, a complete bath and necessary cleaning of his wounds. At first he was frightened and bitter because he had no occasion to trust us, especially after we had cut his hair; their enemies wore their hair short. He was frightened, too, by the necessary, but seemingly harsh, treatment of his wounds. Lee had wounds in his right side, and his left leg had been amputated before he came to us. Under the constant care of the nurses and corpsmen, Lee's right foot improved until he was able to wear a new shoe. It was a big moment for him when the shoes were issued, and he appreciatively gave the left shoe to one of the Korean patients who had befriended him when he was first admitted. Now that friendship had a place, he improved more rapidly. He even sang as he assisted in caring for other patients. Like many other Korean patients, he shed tears and wore a sad expression on the day he left the ship and all the new friends he had made.

Approximately every three months a ship returned to Japan, and the wounded were transferred to a hospital ashore. All personnel were granted a well-earned leave, which we called "R and R" (rest and recreation). In those happy and carefree days we temporarily forgot all the tragedies of war. Then it was back to work again!

One warm and tranquil day we entered Inchon harbor. The sun shone down on us from the blue sky. For a moment one was almost inclined to dream, "The world was at peace again." But we were quite disillusioned when darkness fell and the sky had a crimson mist from anti-aircraft fire.

Our ship was not equipped at this time with a stationary flight deck to accommodate helicopters. Through the ingenuity of our commanding officer, a pontoon barge moored to each side of the ship served as landing platforms for the "whirlybirds," as they buzzed in from the frontlines with their burdens. Call to "Flight Quarters" at first was a novelty. But soon it came to mean more Bunker Hill casualties—our Marines. Bunker Hill in Korea has no association with the famed Boston landmark. It is located northeast of Panmunjom and derives its name from the elaborate bunker system devised by the Communists.

One morning a wounded man was taken from the flight deck to the operating room within a few minutes of his arrival on the ship. At the same moment the operating room nurse arrived. The patient, apparently in extreme shock, was still dressed in battle attire, lying on a field stretcher. Examination revealed severe wounds along his entire right side with the exception of his head. The arm and leg were more severely wounded than the torso because of his bullet-proof vest. An intravenous of blood plasma was given at once, and at the same time the anesthetist was giving oxygen. The operation itself was delayed 35 minutes because of the patient's critical condition. Then came the operation—amputation of his right arm and debridement of numerous scattered wounds on his torso and right leg. His right leg was to be amputated as soon as his strength would permit the operation to be performed.

Two days later, his first request was for the nurse to write his mother a letter.

> Dear Mom,
> I just wanted you to know that I'm OK and that they are taking fine care of me here on the hospital ship. This will be a shock to you, but I have lost my right arm and probably will lose my right leg. I'll probably be in Oakland at the Naval Hospital in about three or four weeks. Tell Louise that I have a lot to talk over with her . . . . Just talk.

While leading a squad of men the day before he came to us, he had been hit by a mortar blast and had been left bleeding and dying on Bunker Hill. A Navy corpsman found him and stemmed the flow of blood. He was brought by helicopter to our ship.

"I'm all right, nurse, don't worry. I don't need anything." Never a complaint, never a whimper was heard. His voice saddened for a moment when he said, "I hope Mom doesn't feel too badly about this. Louise sure loves to dance."

The long awaited day finally arrived. We were going home. Nine long months had passed. We would soon be seeing the Golden Gate, gateway to the U.S.A.

The majority of the medical staff and ship's company had orders to other stations. Some were returning to civilian life. Only a few of us remained that night to hear: "Taps, taps, lights out. All hands turn into your bunks—keep silence about the deck. The smoking lamp is out in all living and berthing spaces."

* * *

Angel of the Orient

Shortly after the tragic demise of Benevolence *in August 1950, another of her sisters, USS* Repose, *headed for Korea. Ensign Lura Jane Emery had been assigned to the hospital ship even when the vessel was still in the yard being fitted out. Surprised and thrilled to have been given that coveted assignment even though she was a junior nurse, Emery quickly plunged into her new duties helping to ready* Repose *for action. Despite what she may have heard from veterans who had served in a previous war, nothing could have prepared her for what she encountered when the ship, soon to be nicknamed "Angel of the Orient," pulled into Pusan.*

Pusan was very grim, dark, and bleak looking. The smell was horrendous because of the refugees who just filled the pier. They had no food. They had no clothes. There were no sanitary facilities. There was just a ditch where they relieved themselves. It was just deplorable! We felt so sorry for those people. We soon found they were eating our garbage. The food service officer began keeping food left over from the officer and enlisted mess separate, and we fed them for quite a while until they suddenly disappeared. They must have been moved out of Pusan, or else some of the people in Pusan took them in. It's a scene I'll never forget.

The first day in port, some Army personnel came aboard and informed us that we were going to get patients at noon. Well, at noon they began arriving, and it just went on and on and on twenty-four hours a day, seven days a week. They were dirty and very sick, but even though the patients were in pain, they were happy to be aboard ship because they knew they were in a safe area. We immediately saw that each patient was bathed, fed, medicated, and prepared for surgery. As soon as they were physically able to go to surgery, they went.

There were American Marines and Army troops, Turks, British, some Australians, but not many South Koreans. There were also a few North Korean POWs who had to be guarded until they could be removed. Basically, most of our patients were UN troops.

The Turks were an interesting group. They were very tough and didn't want any anesthesia when we put sutures in, removed them, or changed dressings or casts. They never flinched. They just told the doctor to do what he had to do. The only problem we had with them was their habit of getting shaving cream and toothpaste mixed up. Because toothpaste and shaving cream came in tubes, they'd use toothpaste to shave and shaving cream to clean their teeth. The corpsmen tried to get them straightened out but never could. Nevertheless, the Turks were a great bunch of fellas to take care of. They were so appreciative. Nothing fazed them. They'd eat whatever you gave them and you didn't have to worry about pain. When we removed dressings, it could be very painful but that didn't bother them. They just told the doctor to go ahead. The doctors would say, "Well, he's a Turk. We don't have to give him any anesthesia; he can take this."

I was on the neurosurgery ward where there were a lot of head injuries and anything that had to do with the spine, the nerves, or the head. Many patients had shrapnel in their brains which had to be removed.

We worked long hours, sometimes twenty-two hours a day. You were lucky if you could get back to your stateroom at 1, 2, or 2:30 in the morning. And then you didn't go to bed. You just took your shoes off and lay across the bed until the Chief Nurse woke you up in the morning and said another train had just come in. This was usually around 6:30. Then you'd get up and start the day over again.

The trains usually came to Pusan at night because of the danger of being bombed during the day. We then went all day but had a lull in the procedures at night around dinner time when there was an opportunity to eat. I then usually showered, put on a fresh uniform, and got ready for another day's work.

There was one patient in particular I'll never forget. He was a young fella with light hair who had been a prisoner of war. The enemy had tied him to a tree and shot at his eyes so he was blind. I don't know the details of how he was freed, but he came in with a group that had been behind the lines as POWs. He wasn't with us very long. Capt. [Russell] Blood, our neurosurgeon, was very good with him. He sat and talked to him a long time, and then they got him out fast and back to the States because there wasn't really much we could do for him on the ship.

About that time, I got body lice from another POW. I thought he had a terrible urticaria [skin eruptions]. I didn't know it was moving urticaria. When I cut his clothes off, I just threw them under the bunk. Later on, a corpsman went through the ward and gathered up all the dirty clothes. What a time I had trying to get rid of those body lice. The problem was that they got into the mattress. Finally, one of the petty officers and the chief nurse decided the only thing to do was to put the mattress in the autoclave and sterilize it with steam. One night I'd sleep on the lower bunk whose mattress had been steamed, and the next night I'd sleep in the upper bunk. I'd switch bunks night to night. Every time I slept in a bunk, they would autoclave the mattress to get rid of the body lice. I was so busy I didn't have time to think about it during the day, but if I sat down to do charting during quiet hour from 1 to 2, I'd feel those things moving all over me. It was miserable. The EENT doctor made rounds in the morning since the neurosurgeon was in the operating room. He'd say to the new patients, "Don't get near that nurse. She's got body lice." Then they'd all whoop and howl. The word got around that the nurse down on neurosurgery had their lice. Anyone who could walk or even get down there on crutches would come see who the nurse was. It really got to be a stress-reliever.

We were unaware of what was going on out there on the battlefield because we were so busy taking care of patients. No one had time to brief us as to what was going on. We had no idea enemy troops were so close to us.

Occasionally, as I went about my work, I'd hear patients talking to one another about what was going on in the field. They would talk about who had been killed and how difficult it was. We were so busy, there wasn't time to sit down and talk to them individually. And we had such a turnover. The patients came in, we got them ready for surgery, they had surgery, and out they went, usually air-evaced to Yokosuka or straight back to the States.

There were times I had two wards, the neurosurgery ward and the general surgery ward next to me. There were patients who had been hit with napalm on that general surgery ward. The damage that had been done was just unbelievable. Napalm is a sticky, jelly-like substance that burned right down into the tissue. There was no medical protocol for taking care of those patients so the doctors had to use their best judgment. I felt so sorry for those patients because they had such burning pain. We gave them narcotics to relieve the pain, and they stayed with us until they were physically able to be sent back to the States. I often wonder about some of them. Did they make it once they got back?

In November [1950] we left Inchon on a special mission to evacuate patients from Chinnampo. When we got there, we had to swing around the anchor for four or five days before heading upriver. There was an Australian chopper pilot who later told us the Chinese were lined up on both banks of the Chinnampo River with their guns ready to fire. The miracle is they watched us go up the river but never fired on us. At night, when we were swinging on the anchor, the captain put a guard on the rail. The whole time we were in Korea and moving around, the ship was blacked out because the Chinese and North Koreans did not honor the Geneva Accords.

What I remember most was how cold it was up there. We took on all these patients with their personal gear plus their ammunition and guns, which were stored down in the hold. We had so many patients and so much gear we couldn't leave until we got a high tide. With our draft, there wasn't enough water to get us down the river.[5]

* * *

Haven Anesthesiologist
After "yard time" on the West Coast for routine maintenance and sometimes major refitting, such as the installation of helicopter landing decks, the three

mercy ships would take on new crews and return to action in Korea. One of Nell Harrington's successors was Dr. Robert Harvey. Another product of the Navy's V-12 training program, Harvey had attended the University of Buffalo (New York) Medical School as a member of the Naval Reserve. He had finished his internship and was just beginning his second year of residency in anesthesia when he heard from the Navy "inviting" him to report for active duty. One day after completing his residency, he received orders to the Chelsea Naval Hospital in Boston. Four months later he was assigned to new duty aboard USS Haven. *It was the end of 1952.*

I was impressed with the size of the hospital ship but wasn't overwhelmed by it. I was also impressed by the personnel—twenty-seven physicians and twenty-seven nurses. All specialties were represented on the medical staff. We had a full functioning ship with good operating rooms, a good blood bank, good anesthesia machines, and good equipment to work with. It was pretty close to the most modern hospital ashore. We weren't compromising at all.

The ship sailed across to Japan, to the Naval shipyard at Yokosuka, and then from there through the Shimonoseki Straits and over to Inchon where we were based.

We were close enough that we could see bombs bursting and flashes of light from gunfire. If there was to be a big push, we'd get ready for a bunch of casualties who would come by train into Inchon, and then be brought by boat out to the hospital ship.

A lot of fresh casualties came in by helicopter right from the aid stations. If they came aboard that way, we had a triage team to meet them right on the helicopter deck. From there they were put on a cart and taken into the operating suite, or they could be triaged and taken to a ward. Then they came to surgery whenever it was indicated. If they just had wounds that had to be closed, and it wasn't a true emergency, they might be scheduled for that afternoon or the next day; it was a twenty-four-hour operation.

Sometimes a lot of casualties arrived at once. One afternoon we did twenty-six cases of secondary closures in two operating rooms. Most of those patients had multiple injuries. Usually we had two operating rooms going at once and sometimes three. That was possible because of our two trained anesthesiologists, one other doctor who had done anesthesia in general practice, and our nurse anesthetist.

Our usual anesthetic was [sodium] pentothal, nitrous oxide, oxygen, and a muscle relaxant. I favored succinylcholine chloride (Anectine) and maybe some narcotics for maintenance. I don't recall using ether, which was explosive. We tried to stay away from explosive drugs.

Most of the time we were available in the operating suite for whatever was needed, but occasionally we'd be asked to come up on deck to intubate a patient or help with a patient who wasn't breathing properly. But it was not our assignment to go out and meet the helicopters when they landed on the flight deck.

We saw a lot of shrapnel injuries from "bouncing bettys," and I can recall specifically some bad eye injuries caused by servicemen tripping bouncing betty mines.[6] These mines came up three or four feet in the air and then exploded.

There were also shrapnel and gunshot wounds. I don't recall seeing many injuries from hand-to-hand combat but certainly a lot of bullet wounds and injuries from blasts. We also took care of people who were injured in other ways. I recall one particular incident. A pilot was taking off from an airstrip carrying a payload of napalm, but couldn't get airborne and hit a steamroller at the end of the runway. He suffered third-degree burns over most of his body, and even though he was alert and could talk, he couldn't see. Before we could do anything, he began developing cerebral edema. We gave him some morphine, which was all that was required for sedation and pain relief at the time. I don't recall if he lived half an hour or an hour. The one thing I didn't do, which I regret, was to get a personal message to his next of kin.

There were a lot of patients with open chest wounds or brain injuries. I remember one of our internists going out to the flight deck one afternoon at lunchtime to meet a helicopter that was coming in. After it landed, the pilot was rotating it around just a little bit when the man walked right into the tail rotor. It took the front of his face right off. Nobody ate anything after that.[7]

Some of our very young patients had injuries to both eyes and you knew they were going to be blind. Even though things like that were very disturbing, we still helped a lot of people. I had the impression that when a wounded Marine arrived on the hospital ship he felt he was finally safe and was going to be all right. And most of the time they were.

* * *

To Have a Purpose

Lt.(j.g.) Nancy "Bing" Crosby joined the Navy in 1949. "I was very delighted because both of my brothers were in the Navy. One went to the Naval Academy and my other brother served in submarines. Would you believe that? Two brothers in the Navy and I was the only one who went to war."

After two assignments, one at the National Naval Medical Center in Bethesda, Maryland, and the other at Naval Hospital Beaufort, South Carolina, the young officer was assigned to USS Haven. *In addition to her nursing skills, Crosby was both a gifted photographer and a natural chronicler. The following excerpts from her journal provide a forthright, contemporary account of life aboard a Korean War hospital ship.*

2 January 1952

Arrived at the USS "Haven" which was painted white and had several large red crosses fore, aft, port and starboard. We were directed to our quarters and found that we were the first out of a group of 25 new nurses to report on board. Ginny [Virginia Brown] and I live together in a cigar box. These rooms are treasures. She inhales when I exhale. We have upper and lower beds, two desks with drawers above and below, a cubboard [*sic*] and a bird-bath of a sink below a medicine cubboard.

It kills me to think of being in uniform constantly except in our room. Can't even dress leisurely in the ward room.

Confusion ran high for the rest of the day because each nurse must have brought at least two to three chests of gear. I sadly stowed away my civilian clothes, brand new, and set about to unpack. Stewards swore as they carted our gear from one deck to another. It was difficult to believe that we were finally on the ship—like being set down in the middle of a dream, wondering what became of the beginning.

7 January

This is the big day for we sail at 1300. The ship is buzzing with activity and all hands eagerly at their noon meal with relish, wondering if that would be the last meal for awhile that they would enjoy.

Up anchor. Two tugs pulled us out of Pier 2 as all hands stood at quarters outside. We circled San Francisco Bay several times, checking our compass. We then started out, passing under the Oakland-Bay Bridge, past Treasure Island, Alcatraz and with San Francisco to port and Oakland to starboard. T'was calm in the harbor but after passing under the Golden Gate Bridge, our luck changed. Was fascinated watching many seals swimming on either side of the ship. The rocky cliffs of the Pacific coast looked cold and lonely.

Stood outside until my teeth began to chip with the intense cold. It would be a long time before we would see the states again and I wanted a mental picture to carry me through the many days at Pusan.

Three nurses are already green and it's a sad sight indeed to look around the table and compare the various shades of white and green. Not too many nurses have ever seen the ocean before, let alone be out in it. We were running 16 knots and the sea was made up of long high swells. It rained the first night and the ship rocked to every conceivable angle.

Movies in the men's ward-room. 10% of the nurses are nursing sea-sickness in their beds. Hope my Crosby luck holds out.

Crosby's luck did hold for the remainder of the voyage. The Maryland native, who had spent her childhood summers sailing Chesapeake Bay, never shared the fate of her "landlubber" colleagues.
When Haven *docked at Yokosuka, Japan, on 23 January 1952, some of the crew had a well-deserved liberty ashore. Everywhere was evidence of what awaited them.*

23 January
This so-called forward area is teeming with activity. Several carriers, the "Valley Forge" alongside, are being supplied and refitted for the Korean campaign. Also several other tankers, destroyers, tenders and various landing craft are swinging at anchor in the bay. It was an impressive sight coming in this morning.

28 January
We departed for Pusan today. Left Pier #11 at 0930 and tied up at a buoy outside the breakwater until 1400. We must go thru "Bungo Suido" Straits during daylight for there are so many islands and the way is crooked.

31 January
We passed through the straits with Moji on port and Shimonoseki on starboard. About 5 large steel-mills were plainly visible and were the backbone of steel production for Japan during World War II. The mountains are extremely rugged and high. The straits were very narrow and a few sunken hulls were still being salvaged from the war. Chinese junks were everywhere, along with a steady stream of UN tankers going and coming from Korea.
Welcome to Pusan. The harbor was full of supply ships and small ships of the line. The "Jutlandia," Danish hospital ship and the USS "Consolation" were tied up together at one pier, and a hot Negro Army band played "If I Knew You Were Coming, I'd 'a' Baked a Cake." "St. Louis Blues," etc.

1 February
Received 160 patients from the "Consolation" bright and early this morning, then waved the ship good-bye. She headed for Japan for a well-deserved R&R. She took the sickest patients to Japan.

5 February

Six of the nurses also toured Pusan for the first time. Glad we went before dark or we might not have been lucky enough to return. Poverty, filth, desolation and frightened animals that were once people make up the population. Didn't see any article of food in their stores that we would even feed the pigs. Saw no vegetables, only dead and dried fish, octopus, etc. The odor turned my stomach and the surrounding filth didn't help.

12 February

Watched about eight UN soldiers being hoisted up on litters this evening. It's like a shot in the arm to see those faces as they first see the ship. It reminds you that you have a purpose if you are inclined to forget.

14 February

Found that the little Korean children, hardly clothed for warmth, picked over the trash and garbage carried from the ship each day. Oh God, give us strength and the will to find the answer.

24 February

Another Sunday in Korea and wasn't able to attend church. However, the sights seen on duty do more to kindle a slightly used soul than do the sermons. These boys are flown from the front in a matter of hours after injury and their fight is transposed from the fight of battle to the fight for life just as rapidly. Their spirit is rarely seen elsewhere. After speaking with them and caring for them, many is the time that I have turned away to hide the tears of gratitude. I marvel at their will to recover. One 20-year-old boy with one leg amputated, and the possibility of losing another before long, plus a bullet wound in his chest and shrapnel in his arm, with hardly the strength to lift his good arm, gave me the biggest wink and smile today. So much can be gained in this nightmare if one can think less of himself and more of others.

Spring 1952 was a season of tension and unrest. The on again-off again truce talks at Panmunjom coexisted with the continuing stalemate along the 38th Parallel. One of the sticking points for the seemingly fruitless negotiations was the repatriation of prisoners of war. It was an issue suddenly magnified by a bloody communist uprising at the Koje-do prisoner of war camp. Across South Korea opposition was also growing to President Syngman Rhee's repressive rule. Lawlessness and violence were on the upswing in cities and villages, with UN personnel often the targets. Communist guerrillas frequently took advantage of the unwary. For Nancy Crosby and her fellow Haven *colleagues, feeling threatened became the norm. And with a rhythmic stream of casualties arriving on the pier at Pusan, the war was never far away.*

27 April

Today we had our first beach-party picnic. Five officers and four nurses crawled into the back of the pick-up and headed north. We passed the UN cemetery, [then] K-9 and pulled up on the north side of the ammunition depot.[8] Just two miles north, four soldiers had been killed on guard duty by Red guerrillas, so we cared not to venture further. We found a beach and pitched camp. We soon had tenderloin steaks cooking over charcoal using Dad's technique without salt. We had two guards standing nearby to keep snipers out of the area, but it still felt a little uncomfortable being in the midst of block-buster bombs and guards with M1 rifles. If one looked the other way toward the water, it almost looked like the states. Soon we had a few dozen Korean children watching our every movement. The 4-year-olds had babies strapped on their backs. Sure isn't like the states. These people look old by the time they reach their teens.

29 May

Troop movements on Pier #1 have increased tremendously in the past few days. One thousand troops are loaded and unloaded on the "Aiken Victory" [T-AP-188] daily and the ones going home are more bedraggled perhaps, but certainly happier than the green boys on their way to the front. The colored band plays hot "shipping over" music to each group but it doesn't lighten the heavy feeling in the pit of one's stomach when the boys are crowded into weapons carriers on the field to a camp nearby. The replacements are noisy but the loudness doesn't cover up the undercurrent of fear. I only wish that they could all be on their way home instead of just beginning the challenge.

30 May

All liberty restricted to Pier #1. Gas masks were issued to all patients and personnel aboard today and I must say that they are weird attachments. I resemble something from Mars wearing one. The officers are wearing side-arms when leaving the ship. I wonder if the next step is to make "Annie Oakleys" out of the nurses.

Two more American GI's were killed near K-9 today while walking through a small Korean village.

17 June

K-9 and the ammunition dump blew up today and several doctors and corpsmen are over there now to aid the wounded. No one knows how many casualties yet and it still is going strong with tremendous fires and explosions.

Following a trip to Japan for refitting and "R&R" for the crew, Haven *returned to Korea in the middle of July. This time the ship anchored off Inchon, a port with a notorious reputation for treacherous tides. Nevertheless, the crew found the change of scenery a welcome respite from squalid Pusan. Within days, the hospital ship's commanding officer solved the problem of transporting patients to the ship. Shutterbug Nancy Crosby recorded that innovative solution on film.*

22 July

INCHON. We landed, or rather dropped anchor at 1530 after a two day trip from Pusan. We are three miles offshore and have a view of the beautiful surrounding water and rocky islands. This seems like a strange place after Pusan because there is so much more activity and pleasant surroundings. The tide drops from 18 to 30 feet depending on the season and the current runs between 5 and 8 knots. At low tide the mud flats can be seen stretching 1½ miles away from the shore. The big guns can be heard from the front 25 miles away, and can be seen at night just north of us. The "Repose" is here, but is very anxious to go to Japan while we are here to relieve her.

"Fleet Acts [Activities]" has supplied us with two large flat barges to be used as flight decks for helicopters and it's so exciting to see them land and take off. We have no aft helicopter landing deck.

25 July

Mother [Eleanor] Harrington had a helicopter ride yesterday, along with two other nurses, and it is hoped that the rest of us can also have a ride in the near future. I shot an entire roll of colored film yesterday of the "egg-beaters" experimenting with our flight deck.

26 July

Six nurses, including me, and three doctors were taken to Seoul via the Marine Corps general's staff car. We found most of the city bombed out with only skeletons of buildings left, bullet holes splattered over the remains. We visited St. Marys cathedral—itself unmarred but the surrounding structures completely destroyed—the Capitol and Sigmund [*sic*] Rhee's home. Had my first helicopter ride and after we were in the air, was informed that the copter's tail assembly had fallen off 7 months ago, and they were trying it out for the first time.

18 August

Yesterday, seven nurses, including yours truly, were invited to visit three of the medical aid companies. Two Marine copters flew down to the ship and we left at about 1100 for "A" med, six miles from the front. We received a royal welcome everywhere and no one seemed to notice our dusty shoes and wet uniforms. It was 110 in the shade. "A" med was similar to the others, made up entirely of tents and included everything absolutely necessary. The O.R. was in a tent with prefab glass between the two tent layers. Had lunch there, then all of us piled into four jeeps escorted by an equal number of doctors and headed north to "E" med. The camp site was similar and we were escorted through the various wards. The beds were only stretchers with blankets over them and the patients, who usually wear nothing, had put on P.J.'s for our benefit. Someone was playing "South Pacific" over the loud speaker and I believe that the boys were pleased to see females again. . . .

We left for "C" company med. Bat., 3 miles from the front. Eleven patients had just been received there and the operating room was a bee-hive of activity. We all walked up to the copter landing on top of a hill and watched an air attack about 5-6 miles away. American bombers were dropping bombs on the communists for about 10 miles along the front and the big clumps of smoke could easily be seen. The noise was very noticeable and it seemed so strange to be that close to the Reds.

Haven *departed Korea a week later for needed maintenance and the installation of her helo deck. On 14 October 1952, as she passed under the fog-shrouded Golden Gate Bridge, diarist Crosby meditated on her recent deployment and safe return. "I had to swallow many times to hold back tears of gratitude." It was a short interlude. On New Year's Day 1953, she reported back aboard* Haven *for her second return to the war zone. Crosby remained in Korea until June, a month before the signing of the armistice.*

Notes
[1]Civilian harbor pilot, Capt. Glenn Havens, also died aboard the rescue tug.

[2]Wooden ships up through the nineteenth century were constructed with frames perpendicular to the keel and spaced from stem to stern. Because these frames were numbered consecutively, it was customary to associate a location aboard ship with the closest frame number. Numbered frames continued when steel eventually replaced wooden hulls.

[3]Because *Benevolence* had suffered such extensive damage and rested on her side, raising the vessel was not an option. In August 1952, the Army Corps of Engineers blew her up as a hazard to navigation.

[4]The two Haven-class ships that remained in mothballs were *Tranquillity* (AH-14) and *Sanctuary* (AH-17).

[5]*Repose's* most heroic performance took place during the hectic fighting days following Chinese intervention in the war. After departing Inchon on 19 November 1950, the ship arrived the next day at the port of Chinnampo, Pyongyang's seaport, and took on many UN casualties, fresh evidence of the Chinese offensive's ferocity. Eight days later the hospital ship inched her way 30 miles upriver through a shallow, rocky channel. The most perilous part of the task was steering the narrow, winding course without running aground. The main channel was so heavily mined that the vessel was forced to proceed up a side channel only twenty-six feet deep in sections at high tide. The *Repose* drew twenty-six feet, six inches. At times the fathometer read the same as the ship's draft, indicating just inches between her keel and the bottom. A helicopter hovered ahead, barely above the water, guiding the vessel and looking for mines.

Her mission successful, *Repose* returned to Inchon on 2 December 1950, having taken aboard more than 750 wounded UN troops before they would have been trapped by the huge communist assault. The rescue was conducted so smoothly and swiftly that it went virtually unnoticed.

[6]An antipersonnel mine that discharged a 75mm shell to about head height before exploding.

[7]The fatal casualty was Lt. Richard B. Hull, MC, USNR.

[8]K-9 was the code number for the airfield at Pusan.

"Whirlybirds"

*M*uch of Korea is a tangle of craggy, forbidding mountains, steep slopes, and narrow, twisted valleys. The snow and ice of the Korean winter made movement even more perilous along tracks often masquerading as roads. In such a hostile environment, the chain of medical evacuation was a nightmare. Moving casualties from the battlefield to aid stations, field hospitals, or eventually a hospital ship required many hours of manhandling and brutalizing discomfort for a patient aboard a stretcher, jeep, and ambulance. What transpired during the Chosin campaign is a case in point. If survival depended upon reaching medical care quickly, the patient's odds were not favorable.

Igor Sikorsky had experimented with an invention in the late 1930s and perfected it by the mid-1940s—the helicopter. The helo truly marked a new era in medical evacuation because it was more efficient and could land virtually anywhere. In April 1944, an Army Air Force lieutenant, who was piloting an early Sikorsky YR-4, performed the first helicopter medevac in Burma. But it wasn't until Korea that the "whirlybird" reached its full potential.

Two companies, Sikorsky and Bell, monopolized the military inventory during the Korean War. Although model number designations differed among the Army, Navy, Air Force, and Marine Corps, the basic airframes and engines were the same. The most recognizable of the Korean War helicopters, the Bell HTL series (Navy), was a three-seat aircraft distinguishable by its Plexiglas bubble canopy, a fabric-covered wooden main rotor, open lattice tailboom, and landing skids. With litters attached to these skids, each helo could carry two patients and, occasionally, more injured. During the first six months of the war, Bell helicopters transported 618 casualties. By the end of 1951, Bell H-13D (Army) and HTL-4 (Marine Corps) helos had evacuated more than 8,500 casualties.

The larger Sikorsky HO3S (Navy) series was a four-seat general utility helicopter. First flown in 1946, it also was the first helicopter used in Korea. The HO3S was not originally equipped with litters, but it was soon retrofitted by having the right window removed and fittings installed to hold a stretcher. With this arrangement, the patient's foot stuck out about eighteen inches through the window. The HO3S carried a pilot and a corpsman, and, as pods were mounted on the fuselage, two *patients could be carried externally. These pods eventually had removable lids installed that protected patients from wind, weather, and rotor wash.*

The HO5S-1 was a three-seater. Two crewmen sat side by side up forward with room for one or two passengers aft. Two stretchers could be carried fore and aft inside the cabin in place of the left side seats.

The Marine HRS-2 or Navy HO4S-1 was a general utility helicopter that could carry a maximum of three litter patients within the cabin. During the latter part of the war, this helo became one of the most popular models.

Early in the war, helicopters helped pinpoint enemy troop concentrations and rescued downed pilots. It was just a matter of time before they would be snatching the wounded from the battlefield and landing them aboard the three hospital ships. This new evacuation system could take place within sixty minutes, the "magic hour" that often meant life or death.

* * *

Birth of the Helo Deck

The name Joel T. Boone is legendary in the Navy Medical Department. By the time he retired from government service in 1955, Vice Adm. Boone had earned the Medal of Honor for valor on the Western Front during World War I, become White House physician for three presidents, and served on Adm. William Halsey's staff as Third Fleet medical officer during World War II. Following Japan's capitulation, Boone was the first Navy physician to enter Japanese prisoner-of-war camps with orders to liberate Allied survivors. Even today, Dr. Boone remains the Navy's most decorated medical officer.

In September 1950, following the successful Inchon operation, Boone, accompanied by an aide and long-time associate, Cmdr. Allen Bigelow, MSC, headed to Korea to assess the state of Navy medicine's support of UN operations. After a good night's sleep aboard USS Rochester *(CA-124), Boone went ashore to find Inchon virtually destroyed. He was also shocked to find tremendous numbers of wounded, mostly South Korean civilians and defeated North Korean soldiers. To Boone's practiced eye, what seemed most lacking was a quick and efficient evacuation system that could move casualties from where they were injured to advanced medical care in the shortest possible time. The presence at Inchon of the hospital ship USS* Consolation *(AH-15) was comforting, but getting patients aboard was problematic. Because of the continuing enemy presence, the white ship had to remain out of artillery range and too far offshore from where she was most needed. Dr. Boone tells the story of how all that changed.*

Enemy wounded and the wounded of our American forces were brought to the beach landing area in Inchon. The roads were becoming very heavily congested with various forms of transportation hurrying in both directions. There were many, many wounded being conveyed to the landing down on the waterfront.

I recognized that the progress of evacuating wounded was very retarded under such circumstances. If relief was not forthcoming expeditiously, many of the wounded would die who had a chance to live otherwise, and the wounded conditions would be aggravated. I knew something had to be done to speed up evacuation of casualties, both American and the enemy—North Koreans. Also a multitude of civilians had been wounded, and relief should be effected for them as quickly as possible.

Bigelow and I returned to the *Rochester* in midafternoon of September 18. I told [Vice Adm. Arthur D.] Struble[1] of my observations and deep concern. I observed that the hospital ship *Consolation* was too far removed from beach landings. He said they were about six miles down the bay and could not be brought up closer because the firing at night on our ships was so intense that we might lose the only hospital ship we had there [*Consolation*] and then be without any. I told Struble that I wished to visit the *Consolation* and inquired how I could get aboard her, except at the expense of a great deal of time.

He said that he could loan me his fastest boat, which would take from an hour to an hour and a half to go from the *Rochester* to the *Consolation*. I knew I would need about an hour aboard the hospital ship to see the patients and confer with the commanding officers, that is, of the ship and of the hospital part of the ship. I did not see how I could make the round trip and accomplish my mission in less than approximately three hours.

It was almost midafternoon when he and I were having our conference about my trip to the hospital ship. Struble said that they would bring me back to the *Rochester*, with exposure to possible fire, after sundown, and no boats were allowed to be under way in Inchon waters after sundown. He did not believe the trip could be made under those conditions as enumerated.

I asked him if there weren't some other way for me to get to the hospital ship. For example, did he have a helicopter aboard?

Struble looked very surprised and said, "Why, yes, I have one on the fantail of the ship."

I asked if I could talk to his pilot.

He said, "Certainly," so he sent for his pilot and I talked to him in Struble's cabin. I asked the pilot if he were willing to fly me down to the hospital ship, and he said he certainly would, but I had to remember that there were no landing facilities on the hospital ship; however, he said I could be lowered from the fuselage of the helicopter by a steel guy wire using a controlled hydraulic pulley. I said it would be a novel trip for me and prove of much value, I was sure.

I told Al Bigelow he did not have to accompany me if he didn't wish to do so; but if he did, it would require two trips of the helicopter from the *Rochester* to the hospital ship and return, because the helicopter only carried a pilot and places for two passengers in the cockpit. A mechanic [assistant crew chief] had to make the trip with us, handling the lowering and hoisting lines for whoever would make the landing and be returned to the helicopter. It was arranged that I would fly first with the pilot and the mechanic, and on a subsequent trip Bigelow would do likewise.

After taking off from the deck of the *Rochester*, we flew toward the *Consolation* and circled it from about 300 feet elevation. Due to the masts, the guy lines, antennas, stack, etc., it would appear there would be no place where a passenger could be landed. Looking down, I spotted what I felt was a large enough space near the deckhouse on the fantail. The pilot felt sure he could land me there so he instructed me what to do.

The mechanic and I were sitting on a seat just behind the pilot. A canvas strap was handed to me, which I placed under my arms and which was attached by a snaffle to the arm of a sling and then was swung out from the helicopter's doorway. There was no closed door. Having done this, I so reported to the pilot. He said, "Now take a hold of a rod on the back of my seat and have one of your feet find a rod underneath my seat. Hold firmly to the rod on the back of the seat and with your foot reach out the doorway, and you will find a rod underneath the doorway on which you place your foot."

Having done this, I reported to the pilot that I was holding on to the rod back of his seat and my foot was on the rod under the doorway. He said, "Now release yourself from holding on to my seat and keep your foot on the rod outside the door, and the metal line will be swung out, held tight by a hydraulic control; then take your foot off the rod outside of the doorway."

I said, "And then what?"

He said, "Then you float into space," and I was then aware that that's when you really get your thrill.

Before I left the cockpit, I was told to put on a life preserver and a "Mae West," named for the well-known be-bosomed actress, which would be inflated in case I would be dropped into the water.

As I was swinging around in my descent from the cockpit of the helicopter to the deck of the *Consolation*, I felt like the man on the flying trapeze and thought of my wife and what her comments would be on my undertaking such an expedition. I thought she would be thinking to herself, "What a fool her old admiral husband was to undertake such a mission."

There was great excitement at seeing my arrival. Many cameras appeared, as they wanted to see this undertaking I had embarked upon. I was pleasantly greeted and escorted to the sick quarters to see patients. I knew time was a very important factor, so I did not delay too long over beyond what I thought would be necessary to accomplish my mission. I saw most of the patients and talked to many of the staff members in addition to the commanding officer of the ship and the commanding officer of the hospital part of the ship.[2]

In returning to the place on which I had landed on the deck, I signaled to the helicopter pilot to pick me up. He sent down on the guy line a life preserver and a Mae West. These I put on and signaled that I was ready to be hoisted aboard. As I was hoisted from the deck and came nearer and nearer to the helicopter, I naturally, because of my weight, spun faster and faster, and, when I was hauled up near the door I had to, as I had been instructed, make a grab for the door frame and pull myself into the cockpit. I missed the doorway by not being able to grab it three times before I successfully got myself into the cockpit area. It was a big relief to be safely back in the cockpit.

Before leaving the hospital ship, Captain Baker, the commanding officer of the hospital part of the ship, asked me to fly over and around the ship before I departed toward the *Rochester*, so that they could get pictures of me in flight. This we did, and then made our successful flight [back] with a feeling of relief that our mission had been successfully accomplished.

Admiral Struble and, I think, most all officers and many of the members of the crew were out to see this expedition return. I thought [they] were apprehensive that we would not safely return.

Having been greeted by Admiral Struble, I asked if I could come into his cabin. I wished to talk to him. I should have said [previously] that before I began to be hoisted from the deck of the *Consolation*, flying around the hospital ship two or three times, and then landing on the *Rochester*, I happened to look at my watch. The consumed time to make that entire trip was ten minutes.

As soon as Struble and I entered his cabin, I said, "Why not build a landing platform on the fantail of the hospital ships for helicopters to land thereon?"

Struble thought I was crazy as hell, he said, for even proposing such a screwball idea. I said no doubt many people thought I was at times, but in this instance I certainly was not. I felt my proposal was a very sound and practical measure.

He said, "I'll prove to you, Joel, how crazy you are." Thereupon he sent for his engineer officer, Rear Admiral George Henderson.

Struble then narrated to Henderson my proposal. Instead of his agreeing with him, Henderson said, "Hell, why didn't we line officers think about it instead of some medical officer! It certainly is a practical idea."

His observation naturally was a surprise to me, but was very gratifying. I knew the proposal, if it were carried out and the provision made on hospital ships, would greatly speed the evacuation of wounded and innumerable lives would be saved. As a result, it was recommended that landing platforms be built on hospital ships. I was pleased to learn later that Vice Admiral Struble and Rear Admiral J.H. Doyle [Amphibious Force Commander] favored the installations.

* * *

Following her participation in the Inchon Invasion and operations at Wonsan and Hungnam, Consolation *was selected as the experimental hospital ship to be fitted with a helicopter flight deck. The ship returned to the naval shipyard at Long Beach, California, where, during a three-month layover, a sixty-foot by sixty-foot landing platform was installed on her fantail. The new platform had a safety net along the sides and after end, with tie-down straps and wooden wheel chocks to help secure the helicopter in rough weather. Two portable windsocks, which could be illuminated, provided pilots a much appreciated landing aid.*

Back in Korean waters in December 1951, Consolation, *now the first hospital ship equipped with a helo deck, was ready to receive patients. She anchored off Sokcho-ri, 15 miles above the 38th Parallel, and took her first patient aboard by helicopter on 18 December.* Consolation *had inaugurated a new era in patient care on that date. Crewman Pearce Grove was there the day Dr. Boone's concept became reality.*

First Helo Landing

I don't know exactly how the idea came about for installing a helo pad on the ship. However, there was talk of that as we left Inchon en route around the peninsula to Wonsan. When we left Wonsan and returned to the States, the purpose was to install the helicopter pad, and the *Consolation* was the first to have it done.

We were in the Long Beach shipyard where construction took just about two months. The construction on the fantail was fantastic. The helo pad was quite large, and we were all amazed how they could get it on there. It was a superstructure welded right onto the ship and built up so that nothing interfered with the landing and takeoff of the helicopters. The deck of the helicopter pad was wood. The job was done as quickly as they could possibly get it done. I witnessed the trials for the helicopter landings with the new helo deck in the ocean just outside of Long Beach, but they were very short. There didn't seem to be any problems whatsoever. It worked just fine, and soon we were on our way back to Korea. The idea was to get back as quickly as possible, and we made use of the new deck just before the Hungnam evacuation.

I remember the very first landing. Everyone aboard ship tried to observe it because it was so historic. This was why we went all the way back to the States in the middle of a war to get this put on the ship. Then to see it actually put into operation was very exhilarating and very impressive. The percentage for saving life went skyrocketing. It was such a lifesaving concept. It was really something to see the helicopters come in and land and the patients taken right off and brought directly to operating rooms. We knew we were seeing something new and we thought, "Oh, my gosh, this is marvelous!" They were coming virtually from the battlefield to the operating room. I remember talking to many patients who thought that this was heaven on earth.

There were many times when the seas were rough and it was difficult landing the helicopters. You also had to be careful taking them off. The landing pad would be going up and down, but it worked. It worked!

* * *

Like a Hen on Her Eggs

Helicopters serving as ambulances soon became the norm aboard Consolation *and then her sister ships,* Haven *and* Repose. *In some cases a patient could be on the operating table less than thirty minutes after incurring an injury on the battlefield. During one communist offensive in September 1952, sixty-two helicopters landed on* Consolation's *helo deck in a single twenty-four-hour period.*

This aircraft also substituted for the traditional method of getting patients aboard. At sea, the breeches buoy was often used for transferring patients between ships. When hospital ships were anchored offshore, patients were brought alongside in small boats—LCVPs (Landing Craft Vehicle and Personnel), LCTs (Landing Craft Tank), or LCMs (Landing Craft Medium). The vessel's electric winch would lower its cable slings to hoist stretchers aboard. However, heavy seas often made this operation less than desirable. Helicopters were not limited by sea conditions that kept small craft in port.

Aboard any of the three hospital ships in port or on station off the Korean coast, the radioman listened intently for messages from incoming helicopters. A Marine Corps reporter for Leatherneck *magazine described one such event aboard* Consolation.

"Hospital ship *Consolation*. This is Charlie Three. I have one walking wounded and two litter cases, one a serious head injury. Will arrive at your ship in approximately three minutes."

Within seconds this message reaches the Officer of the Deck on the bridge. Flight quarters is sounded on the PA system throughout the ship. The Chief of Medicine is notified and he alerts the neurosurgeon. The bugle call "Flight Quarters" brings many men on the double to the flight deck on the stern to prepare for the landing and reception of the wounded. On hand are: the command duty officer, landing signal officer, flight duty doctor for the day, damage controlmen who stand by with firefighting equipment, two chockmen, four litter bearers, a telephone talker to establish communications with the bridge, and the master at arms. A crash boat crew with hospital corpsmen stands by in one of the motor whaleboats in case of an emergency ditching.

In less than sixty seconds word is passed by telephone to the bridge to notify the pilot by radio that he may land. Back on the flight deck the LSO (landing signal officer) stands upwind ready to jockey the helicopter into position with his complicated system of hand signals. The helicopter comes in, hovers over the deck, gently sets down like a hen on her eggs, and cuts its engine.

Before the rotor blades have coasted to a stop, the chockmen have secured the plane in position and the doctor and litter bearers are disembarking the patients. The ambulatory are guided to the hospital spaces while the litters are carried up the ramp to an emergency treatment room for examination and disposition. Total time from shore to ship and treatment, less than five minutes.

The installation of helo decks on Haven *and* Repose *did not follow the conversion of* Consolation *as quickly as the Navy might have hoped. In the interim, there was another solution of getting helicopter-borne patients aboard. As* Haven *lay at anchor off Pusan in the summer of 1952, her commanding officer, Capt. Cyril Hamblett, USNR, borrowed two 50-foot by 146-foot flat barges. These barges had been formerly used by the Army to haul cargo within the port of Inchon. They now moored the wooden decked rafts on either side of* Haven. *Firefighting equipment, wind direction indicators, and warning lights were added, and a painted yellow disk on the deck of each raft marked the landing zone. Litter hoists then lifted patients aboard. During the very hectic period from 26 July to 23 August 1952, helicopters brought some 160 wounded to her floating helo decks.*

* * *

Cavalry from the Sky

Marine sergeant Stavros Moungelis was a helicopter crew chief who arrived in Korea in December 1952. He served there for two years, not leaving for home until seventeen months after the signing of the armistice in July 1953. Headquartered up near the 38th Parallel, his squadron, HMR-161, already had a reputation for getting the job done. One of its choppers had even made the first night landing aboard Repose *in July 1952, carrying a patient from Charlie Medical Company. With Korea's notorious bad roads and severe weather, it was increasingly common for helicopters to ferry supplies and evacuate the wounded. Getting these critically injured men safely out to the hospital ships was something Moungelis will never forget.*

HMR-161 stands for Helicopter Marine Transport Squadron 161. We were part of the 1st Marine Aircraft Wing attached to the 1st Marine Division. It was the same for the other helicopter and aircraft observation squadron—VMO-6. They would take the wounded from the back side of a hill where a battle was raging to a med station. We took them from the med station to the hospital ships. Our helicopters were the HRS-2s made by Sikorsky which replaced the model HRS-1s. Later the HRS-2s were replaced by the first model run of the HRS-3s. Although there were other helicopters used in Korea, such as the Sikorsky HO5S, which was very underpowered, my favorite was the HRS-2, the "workhorse" of the Korean War. Our squadron crest was inscribed "Equitatus Caili" [Cavalry from the Sky].

As a crew chief, I was in charge of the passengers and the load, but we crew chiefs had no [medical] responsibility for the patients we carried. We never had any special training for that.

We were based just east of the 1st Marine Division CP [command post], east of Munsun-yi and south of Panmunjom. There was a main supply route that split our camp. On the north side of the road were tents. On the south side of the road, where there had been rice paddies, we graveled and oiled the area to make helopads. The most helicopters we had at any one time was about fifteen. We had our rear echelon between Inchon and Seoul, a place called Yongdung-po, also referred to as ASCOM City.

We took over what had been a World War II Japanese ammunition factory and converted the ground floor into an office, mess hall, showers, one stall barber, and shops for heavy maintenance—transmission, engine changes, and that type of thing. We turned the second floor into a barracks and the roof into a night movie. The heads were the outdoor type. We were living good, here away from the MLR [Main Line of Resistance].

In a typical month we had thirty medevacs. One month we transported seventy-four casualties to the hospital ships. Sometimes there were up to three ships there in Inchon harbor. Some ships were from Denmark and the Netherlands.

The HRS-2 could carry a maximum of three litter patients internally in the cabin. You could put two on one bulkhead and one on the other. Sometimes, when we just had one patient, we just put him on the deck. Or if we only had two, we could put them on the deck and not even strap the litters into the wall. We would fly with one or two pilots and a crew chief. It was not common practice to bring a doctor or corpsman with the patient on those trips and rarely did we have a corpsman or a doctor who accompanied a patient on our medevacs. I preferred one pilot so I could get some "stick" time flying back home. Most crew chiefs could fly if the situation dictated, including takeoff and landing. I accumulated many stick time hours, as I knew all the sites in our sector. I was used to familiarizing newly assigned pilots to our squadron.

We'd always pick patients up from one of the med stations—Able, Baker, Charlie, and Easy Med. They had been stabilized and were at a point where they could be transported. If these patients had to go by truck and barge to the hospital ship, I don't know what their chances would have been in making it. Although there were medevacs done during the day, they were usually done at night and most of those night flights took place between 8 o'clock and 2 A.M.

A typical day might be something like this. We'd be there standing by awaiting whatever missions came down for the day. We had an operations section with a liaison person, probably an aviator, at the 1st Marine Division headquarters to see what the daily workload would be. The requests were then passed to our squadron operations, and our flight line would then get the word and we would be assigned a mission. We had all kinds of missions. Our main job in Korea was not confined to medical evacuations. We did troops lift, reconnaissance, and rocket launcher flights. There was a period of major floods when we carried supplies that normally would have gone by road. This included bunker materials, sandbags, ammunition, water, rations, all logistics for the 1st Marine Division.

Let's say we got a call for a medevac from Able Med to a hospital ship. We'd fly into Able Med and stay turned up. That is, we didn't shut down the engine. They would be waiting for us and would bring the Marine out on a stretcher. Usually they had one or two patients. Very seldom did we get three at a time. We preferred to have one or two instead of three. That way we didn't have to put one on the wall. If we had two, we'd just place them on the floor. If we had three, we'd hang two on one bulkhead and one on the other using sling hooks attached to the bulkhead. And then there were straps that came down from the middle of the cabin ceiling to hold the one side of the stretcher—front and rear.

Sometimes we had hanging intravenous bottles. There was one occasion—it was a night flight. The patient, as far as I remember, was almost dead. I recall his arm. It was just emaciated; it looked as though he had been on a starvation diet for three months. At night the lighting inside the helicopter cabin was very dim. There was something like a flashlight on the ceiling that you could pull on down on a long cord and direct to read a map or whatever you were doing. But it was not a bright light at all. This Marine had an IV that had been placed in a leg vein. Well, the damn thing had fallen out. I don't think he pulled it out consciously. It looked like it hadn't been taped down properly. I was concerned but glad that we were at least halfway to the hospital ship by this time. I took the needle end of the line and stuck it into the head of his penis. I had heard the penis is a blood vessel. I don't think I could have succeeded inserting it in the arm or leg. I didn't have enough light. I don't know whether that man pulled through or not, but I do know that he was still alive the day after we delivered him.

When we landed aboard that hospital ship the next day with another patient, a doctor came out and said, "Did you come in here last night with a patient that had an IV in his penis?"

I said, "Yes. I did that."

He then said, "You probably saved his life."

If I had to estimate how many wounded I transported from a med station to a hospital ship while I was in Korea, I would guess probably not more than a hundred. That one patient with the needle business was the only one that I had occasion to attend to.

Finding the hospital ship was never really a problem, even at night. On clear nights, the ship was all lit up. You could easily spot it. For bad-weather night flights, they had a big searchlight on the ship and they would just throw it up into the sky. This helped when the weather was bad—cloudy and so forth. We flew in any weather. We were very seldom grounded. It would take a hell of a storm to ground us.

Once we landed, corpsmen and other personnel came out and picked up the patient. And then we were gone inside of five minutes. It took about a half hour to ferry the patients from the med station to the hospital ship. The total mission was about an hour and a half from the time we took off until the time we landed back at our unit.

After the armistice in July 1953, we participated in the prisoner exchange. We transported a lot of the seriously sick and/or wounded POWs to an Army hospital near Seoul. It was very, very sad—horrible. There had been some effort to clean up the American POWs before they were released, but the Republic of South Korean [ROK] prisoners and KMC [Korean Marine Corps] prisoners, who had been held up in the north, were in terrible shape. This was probably the worst sight I've ever seen in my entire life. A lot of them were on stretchers, crutches, or double canes.

Most of the people were able to walk; a few were not, but almost all our released prisoners went by helicopter to an Army field hospital near Seoul for processing. We would take a couple of them at a time. If they were on stretchers, we could take a maximum of three. If they were ambulatory, maybe we could take one or two more, depending upon whether I had one pilot or two. The whole squadron was involved with this. Other South Korean POWs were transported by truck, upon carrier vehicles, jeeps, and field ambulances.

It was a real crazy situation. There was something in the agreement that we must use Indian Gurkha troops to take care of security at the prisoner exchange.

The Gurkhas came to Inchon Harbor by British aircraft carrier, and the deal was that they could not set foot on North or South Korean territory. So the task of transporting these professional soldiers from the British carrier to Panmunjom was up to us, and we transported them by helicopter to neutral no-man's-land.

Around that time there were outbreaks of [epidemic] hemorrhagic fever so we also took patients from the med stations only to that Army hospital near Seoul. The soldiers and Marines I transported were out of it, almost comatose. I understood that if they came out of it in two or three days, they would live. If they didn't, they died. That's all I know about that disease, other than it came from rodents, flies, and mosquitoes that feasted on troops killed on the battlefield, [and these insects and rodents] then bit survivors. To this very day, I take a minimum of three great showers every day!

I know that my service in Korea and later Vietnam was honorable and godly. I prefer to think about the lives I may have saved, as opposed to the lives I know I helped take.

Notes

[1]Struble was Commander 7th Fleet.

[2]Following Boone's visit, Capt. [Robert E.] Baker sent a report to the surgeon general of the Navy, Rear Adm. H. Lamont Pugh. "18 September 1950. Admiral Boone and Commander Bigelow came aboard via helicopter for a short visit and Admiral Boone stated that he would try and arrange for us to move [the hospital ship *Consolation*] closer to the beach since the long boat ride was believed to be detrimental to the patients' welfare. On 21 September our anchorage was shifted to a position off Wolmi do Island, providing a much shorter boat ride for casualties."

8

On the Bomb Line

*W*hen the United Nations first responded to the Korean crisis in 1950, U.S. Navy battleships, cruisers, and destroyers began pounding communist troop concentrations and bombarding enemy roads, railyards, and factories within reach of their guns. Carrier-based aircraft soon added their mobile punch. In fact, by 1952, the U.S. Navy had unloaded more ordnance on North Korea than it had on Japan during all of World War II.

Following surface action and air activity that neutralized North Korea's lilliputian navy early on, wooden-hulled minesweepers went close inshore to clear anchored and floating mines off Wonsan and other harbors. That such duty was perilous is beyond debate. During the war, mines sank five of these craft.

The continuing presence of Navy ships in North Korean waters generated other casualties. Shore batteries occasionally scored hits on their tormentors. During three years of conflict, eighty-seven incidents were reported in which U.S. vessels suffered damage either by striking mines or receiving hostile fire.

Despite the occasional excitement, "cutting furrows in the sea" and maintaining a blockade of the Korean coast described the daily routine of shipboard life. When not chipping paint and swabbing decks, more than a few sailors recall firing at an unseen enemy or scanning the skies for communist aircraft day after day. For those manning sick bays, it was treating colds, sore throats, minor injuries, sprains, fractures, venereal disease, and the occasional appendectomy. Yet, as in any war, everything could change in an instant.

* * *

"Like a Bad Movie"

South Dakotan Clifford Roosa began his military career as a student in the Army's Enlisted Reserve Corps during the early days of World War II. After what he calls a series of fortuitous events, Roosa was transferred to the Army Specialized Training Program in which he studied engineering before being switched to a premed program. He then attended medical school at the University of Rochester, was discharged from the Army in February 1946, and continued medical studies until graduation in 1949 when he joined the Naval Reserve. The following year he *was called to active duty and reported to the Denver recruiting station to examine recruits and recalled Reservists.*

After a stint at an infirmary in Orange, Texas, Roosa received orders to USS St. Paul *(CA-73), berthed in Japan. He then flew to Hawaii, to Midway, and then to Japan, where, on a cold, foggy, February morning in 1952, he "stood on the dock at Yokosuka, Japan, looking up at this huge, gray ship and wondered, 'What would be my fate?'"*

Just days later, the heavy cruiser and its newest officer were on station off Korea's east coast, where her 8-inch guns were needed to support UN troops ashore. The fledgling ship's doctor would soon be called upon to attend victims of one of the war's most catastrophic accidents.

We held sick call daily on the *St. Paul*. Usually it would be most busy on days that we rearmed or refueled. Those days were hard, hard work for the crew. The winters in Japan and Korea are remarkably cold and damp. Working on the main deck in those conditions was something that most people would shun, if possible.

I routinely saw a lot of sore throats, stomach flu, colds, minor injuries, and, occasionally, pneumonia or other serious illness. We also had some experience with venereal disease. Invariably, when there was a general quarters alarm, the crew would hurry to their stations and forget to duck when they went through the hatches. There was a remarkable number who appeared in sick bay with a lunate laceration over an eyebrow. We sewed them up, often without anesthesia—because they were kind of stunned and didn't feel pain—and sent them back to duty.

We had quite a lot of orthopedic injuries—fractures and sprains. Three men fractured their femurs at one time when they fell from the same catwalk above the quarterdeck. There was a lot of seasickness each time we left port. Dramamine was usually helpful, but sometimes we had to admit a patient and hydrate him with intravenous fluids. Prior to boarding, I worried about seasickness myself, but I never experienced this malady.

During my second cruise on the *St. Paul*, we received word that a communication ship run by the South Koreans had a sick person aboard, and requested medical assistance. We pulled alongside and, in heavy seas, I was sent by bosun's chair to do an evaluation. It was apparent that the patient had appendicitis. By this time, the seas were so turbulent that my return with the patient was deemed unsafe. I had been thoroughly doused in the icy water on the way over and concurred in this decision. I placed ice packs on the patient's abdomen and kept an eye on him overnight. The next morning the seas had subsided and we returned to the *St. Paul*. At surgery, the appendix had not ruptured and the patient made an uneventful recovery.

The unusually severe motion of the smaller vessel in the very heavy seas coupled with the permeating odor of Kimchee did not cause me to be seasick.[1] I knew I had it made.

When we did not have a junior officer, or if we were particularly busy, I worked sick call and supervised in-patient care. Later on, as senior medical officer, there was a lot of paperwork and preparation for inspections. I gave many lectures to the crew about health matters, including venereal disease. In my leisure time I studied, but also played bridge, cribbage, and acey-deucy. I gave morning and evening reports to the captain daily.

During my general internship, I had little experience in surgery. I studied my surgical books into the night and with some experience became a passable surgeon. I recall my first appendectomy while the ship was rolling in a heavy sea. We strapped the patient to the narrow table and used ether for anesthesia. Later we used spinal anesthesia when possible because it is generally a safer method.

The next day the patient's name and diagnosis appeared on the sick list. The ship's commanding officer, Capt. [Frederick] Stelter, called me up to his quarters and asked me why I had not informed him of this procedure. It seems I knew very little of Navy protocol and ceremony. I had never even taken an indoctrination course. The Korean War accelerated many assignments. The captain seemed to understand this. He advised me that for all significant medical events he should be notified in person, and for this type of surgery he had to give permission.

The *St. Paul* was cruising an area called the "bomb line" and often involved in shore bombardment. I remember going up to the 02 level one day, which is two levels above the main deck. I opened the hatch and looked out while the 5-inch guns were firing. A volley was fired at a high trajectory and the concussion and sound were incredible. I experienced ringing in my ears for days. Another time, while in Wonsan Harbor, I again became curious. I could hear some unusual activity outside my battle station, which at this time was the captain's quarters. I cracked the hatch, looked out, and there were nearby spumes of water from enemy fire. I thought, "This could be a mistake." I quickly closed the hatch and considered hiding under the captain's bed.

We threw a lot of ammo into North Korea in 1952 and 1953. I'll never forget 21 April 1952. I was in the officers' ward room when I felt and heard a "thump." Somehow I knew that something bad had happened. Perhaps we had been hit by enemy fire. I hurried to sick bay. Soon stretcher bearers brought in two patients. Both were unconscious, their clothing and faces were blackened, breathing was rapid and shallow, pulses were present but very faint. It was apparent that they were in extremis. They both died before we had a chance to begin any specific treatment.

The word came down that there had been an explosion in an 8-inch turret and that there were many more casualties. I went topside to the turret hoping that an early assessment might be helpful but, as each body was delivered, it was obvious that nothing could be done. I can still smell the acrid, searing sensation of burning cordite. We placed all these men on deck and went through the formality of pronouncing them dead. There were thirty dead and no survivors of the turret fire. It was a bad day. We were all kind of numb.

Fortunately, the explosion did not carry to the powder magazine as this would have been a real catastrophe. The victims had died of suffocation, burns, or both, but most had succumbed to suffocation when the explosion deprived the closed space of oxygen. At the same time, the fire and smoke severely injured their tracheas and lungs. Even had they survived the initial explosion, they would not have survived in any case.

I was included in the investigation that followed and gave testimony as to the condition of the victims and the causes of death. I did not know the result of the investigation or if anyone was accountable. I was then appointed as inventory officer and, with another officer, inventoried the private possessions of these thirty men. It was a sad duty.

I don't believe I felt the full impact of the event from a personal standpoint until we delivered the bodies at Pusan. There had been some consideration of burial at sea because we were in battle exercise, but then we received permission to leave the area and transfer the bodies to the hospital ship [*Haven*] at Pusan. We were replaced on the line by the USS *Wisconsin* [BB-64]. As the victims were transferred from the ship, someone played "Taps." The whole thing just seemed like a bad movie. I find it hard to talk about it even now.

* * *

Carrier War

Thirteen U.S. Navy aircraft carriers served in Korean waters as part of Task Force 17—Antietam, Badoeng Strait, Bataan, Bon Homme Richard, Boxer, Essex, Kearsarge, Leyte, Philippine Sea, Point Cruz, Princeton, Rendova, and Valley Forge. Planes flying from their decks had many missions besides providing close air support to UN troops. One was interdiction—destroying enemy roads, bridges, trains, tanks, trucks, and aircraft on the ground. Another important role was combat air patrol—protecting the vulnerable task force from hostile aircraft when its own planes were flying missions over enemy territory.

The carrier war was a dangerous business. Launching ordnance-laden planes and recovering them after their missions required skilled crews. Carriers were, and still are, floating cities, airfields, and fuel depots, and a home to thousands of crewmembers, pilots, and their support personnel.

A carrier hull is also a warren of compartments crammed with steam turbine main propulsion engines, and countless pumps, ventilators, and generators. Korean War-era carriers, like today's nuclear behemoths, maintained machine shops below decks where piston engines and jet engines could be torn down and rebuilt. Steam-driven catapult machinery, a hangar deck which could house more than eighty aircraft, and several weapons magazines were also housed below the flight deck.

Fuel was the lifeblood of these floating airbases. A carrier hauled hundreds of thousands of gallons of oil for its own turbines, and aviation gasoline and jet engine grade kerosene to feed the insatiable appetites of its aircraft.

The aircraft carrier had two medical departments, one to care for the main crew and the other to handle the special needs of the embarked air group, usually consisting of three squadrons. "Sick bay," or main medical, contained an operating room with requisite x-ray facilities, perhaps a small medical laboratory, and a patient ward. Sick bay was usually staffed by three physicians, one having the title of senior medical officer, and perhaps fifteen to twenty hospital corpsmen. As on other naval warships, battle dressing stations were strategically located throughout the vessel. During general quarters, they were manned by physicians, dentists, and hospital corpsmen. The dental department, usually contiguous to sick bay, may have contained two chairs and been staffed by two dentists and two or three dental technicians.

The other sick bay's sole purpose was to care for personnel of the embarked air group. Somewhat smaller than main medical, it was usually located on a level near the hangar deck and flight deck with easy access to the latter. This sick bay near the decks had three flight surgeons, each representing one of the squadrons making up the air group. Several hospital corpsmen supported this smaller medical operation.

The flight surgeon was a specialist in aviation medicine. His training included a wide background of different specialties—EENT (eye, ear, nose, and throat), psychiatry, cardiology, and aviation physiology. Indeed, his preparation for the job also required flight training. It took a pilot to treat a pilot. Although the flight surgeon often diagnosed and treated colds, gastrointestinal maladies, and common injuries, as did his colleagues in the main sick bay, he was always on the alert for inner ear anomalies unique to aviators, such as barotitis or barosinusitis, and other conditions that could affect a pilot's flying status. He also watched for emotional problems and abnormal stress. If the aircraft carrier's entire purpose was to launch and recover aircraft, the justification for the flight surgeon was to ensure the health of that warship's most precious cargo—its pilots.

* * *

Flight Surgeon

Dr. Wayne Erdbrink joined the Naval Reserve in 1942 and went to medical school as an apprentice seaman in the V-12 Program. Still in medical school when World War II ended, he opted to become a regular naval officer and interned at Naval Hospital Philadelphia. Following internship, Erdbrink applied for and was accepted into the flight surgeon program at Pensacola, Florida. Fresh out of medical school and internship, he plunged into those aspects of medicine peculiar to aviation—eye, ear, nose, and throat, cardiology, and psychiatry. He also learned about centrifuges, low-pressure chambers, and soloed in the Navy's SNJ basic trainer aircraft.

Lt. Erdbrink was then assigned duty with two flight squadrons headquartered in Germany. He took part in the Berlin Airlift and returned home with his squadron as part of the Military Air Transport Service that flew regular overseas missions to Europe out of Westover Air Force Base, Massachusetts. He was still doing these runs when he was reassigned to an air group forming in Alameda, California. Air Group 15 would soon deploy to Korea aboard USS Antietam *(CV-36), a Ticonderoga-class carrier that had joined the Pacific Fleet too late to see any action during World War II.*

Antietam had a four-striper in command. The exec, the air boss, and the chief engineer were all regulars, but the rest of the officers and crew members were all Reserve. My air group staff—about six people—were all regulars. Our CAG [commander air group], the administrative officer, the supply officer, the flight operations officer, the disbursing officer, and the medical officer were all regulars. Otherwise, we had four Reserve squadrons—two jet squadrons from New York State, one dive bomber squadron from Illinois, and one Corsair fighter squadron from Denver, Colorado.

I had a chief and six corpsmen. My flight and general quarters station was Repair 8, which was the after end of the island. We had our own small sick bay and aviation examining room on the carrier separate from the carrier's medical department. It was in a different part of the ship where I could have quick access from Repair 8. The chief and corpsmen would hold aviation sick call there. If I were needed, I could duck down. We took care of the air group enlisted and officer personnel separate from the ship's sick bay. Every morning at 0400, I was on the flight deck with two corpsmen, and we were there until the last recovery at 2200 at night.

Most of what I did as a flight surgeon was provide psychological support. It was a family. I visited the ready rooms when the pilots were being prepped for their missions, and I was up on the flight deck at the catapult with the catapult officer for every launch. There I wore a white cloth helmet and sweatshirt with a red cross on them. And everybody knew who I was. I was there when they were launched and when they landed. It was more than hands-on medicine. From my standpoint, aviation medicine was truly camaraderie and friendship.

As part of Task Force 77, we flew combat missions with two carriers. We flew for three days and then refueled on the fourth day. This alternated between carriers so we had that time off to take on ammunition and gasoline, etc. Many of the elective things that had to be done were done on that fourth day. When they did surgery in the medical department's O.R., I was sometimes the amateur anesthesiologist. My colleagues and I were all friendly. We all knew each other and each other's limitations, but we always did what we could do to help each other.

In order to launch jet aircraft, even with the catapult, which was the old steam catapult, we had to have thirty knots of wind over the deck. Much of the time we were in Korea it was winter and there was snow all over the place. I forget what the water temperature was. You dressed in layers. There was a shelter you could duck in to warm up periodically. We were at our flight duty stations either for launch or recovery. We didn't have in-flight refueling back then so the jets would only be up for two hours. The props, however, could be out three to four hours on their missions. Those were the Corsairs and ADs—the dive bombers.

The external ordnance they carried were 500-pounders and 200-pounders. The jets even carried 250s on their wings plus their cannon. The ADs might carry a 1,000- or 2,000-pounder amidship.

In the winter, pilots wore what was called a "poopie suit" that would give them about ten extra minutes of protection in cold water. It was a monstrous rubber thing with boots and gloves that went over everything. The parachute and other gear went over it. Once you got your flight suit on and all this over it, it was bulky to get in the cockpit. The Corsair pilots and the jet pilots had a helluva time.

As I recall, we only had one incident when a plane went in the water. The pilot ejected as soon as he hit the water. With our helicopter always airborne for every takeoff and landing, he was brought out fairly quickly. I remember him now— "Mo" [Aaron Modansky]. He had hemorrhaging into the muscle and cutaneous injuries. He was hospitalized and became the responsibility of the ship's medical department. I just visited him daily to check on his progress. It's amazing that he got back on flying status.

We also had two pilots downed near Wonsan. One ditched and one bailed out. Our helicopter rescued them both and brought them back to the ship. Outside of abrasions, they were both in good shape.

There was one horrendous flight deck accident when I was aboard. A returning Panther jet dived for the deck, missed all the wires, and bounced over the four-foot-high Davis barrier made of nylon. It then hit the parked aircraft up forward and plowed into the tail—the exhaust—of another jet. It was just as though he had flown into a tunnel. There was a chain-reaction collision of aircraft. I was able to find one of the pilot's arms and fingerprint him. Then we buried him at sea in his aircraft. I think we had six flight-deck personnel who were tying down aircraft forward who were also killed. The medical department put out a call for any undertakers aboard to report to sick bay. We suspended flight operations for the rest of the day and night.

I recall another incident. I shared a stateroom with a dive-bomber pilot. We were forward of the hangar deck. A jet's 20mm cannon fired when they were servicing the plane and the shell went right through my bunk. I happened to be sitting there but was leaning over doing something when the shell went right past my head. I sort of heard a bang and then a "pft." And that was it. It was amazing that it did no damage to human or ship.

Even though an aircraft carrier is probably the most dangerous place anyone could be, especially for ordnance people and fuel personnel, we had very few injuries. Everybody was really on their toes and very conscious of safety. It was amazing. Night carrier operations were especially challenging.

Duty as a flight surgeon was special, particularly from a human relations standpoint. You were with a group of pilots you saw every day, heard their complaints in the wardroom, and went on R & R with. When you were aboard ship, there were operations for three consecutive days. You were up at four in the morning 'till eight or ten at night. Then you played poker with them on the third night. They were all wonderful people.

* * *

Pilot in Distress

Lt. Cmdr. Aaron Modansky was already an experienced World War II combat pilot before he reported aboard Antietam *as part of VF-831. During the last campaign of that war, he flew F6F Hellcats. In the intervening years Modansky remained active in the Naval Reserve and transitioned to jets, flying with a reserve squadron out of Floyd Bennett Field, Brooklyn, New York. During that time he learned to fly the new Grumman F9F Panther, and maintained his flying skills by making at least three hundred carrier takeoffs and landings.*

Antietam *arrived off North Korea in the fall of 1951, and her aircraft were soon flying almost daily missions against enemy targets. In January 1952, Lt. Cmdr. Modansky would live every pilot's worst nightmare, a catastrophic mishap on takeoff that nearly cost him his life.*

We flew two types of missions. One was to fly over enemy territory and we did what they called "interdiction." We shot up railroad trains, tanks, trucks, airplanes on the ground; we saw very few airplanes in the air by that time. Their top pilots had been killed and most of the aircraft had been destroyed. So we had superiority in the air. We would destroy their supply lines dramatically.

The other type of mission was the combat air patrol where we flew cover over the fleet while other people were flying missions over enemy territory. We'd put our wings on sideways because when you are on combat air patrol, you fly in a left-hand turn for maybe two hours in a circle.

I'll never forget the day I had my accident. I was having a catapult shot to take off and the aileron controls froze. There were certain ports that were supposed to be cleaned because we were operating in sub-zero conditions and ice would build up. They should have stuck something in there like a pipe cleaner to clean them out but didn't. We know that ice got in because of the way the controls reacted. They just locked up.

I was wearing what they called an "immersion suit," a heavy rubber suit that gave you a few more minutes of protection from the cold if you landed in the icy ocean. Anyway, when I was shot off the catapult, the plane started to roll to the right. That is, the left wing was coming over and the right wing was dipping. Had I continued to let it roll, I would have gone on my back into the water. You're taught to make these split-second decisions, and I knew very well that I didn't want to go in on my back because that would minimize my chances of getting out. We were trained pretty well. So I opted to fly the plane down into the water out of the path of the carrier to the ship's starboard side. I might have achieved 120 or 130 knots at that point.

The impact tore both wings and the tail section off—the whole nine yards. I recall that I didn't panic when I went under. I knew that somehow I had to get to the surface. They say that I tore this heavy duty webbing that would take ten guys on the deck to tear. But, evidently, adrenalin was flowing.

We did a lot of swimming training in our preflight situation. We also trained to get out of an airplane that was inverted underwater and swim away. We learned to swim to the surface, remove your pants, put knots in it, and make a temporary inflatable thing out of it. All that training seemed to help. I also remember having sat on a safety board regarding the death of a guy named Bill Callahan. He was killed in a similar circumstance. He did not have his shoulder harness and his seat belt on tight. So when I knew that I was going in, I flew the plane with one hand and cinched everything tight with the other. I had everything so tight that I couldn't blink. The proof of the pudding is that I'm here.

Anyway, the plane hit and broke into thousands of pieces and I went under. The only thing left was the cockpit going down, and that's what I struggled underwater to get out of. They estimated that I went about thirty feet underwater. The rest of the airplane was completely demolished. Both my legs were paralyzed, and I had a two-and-a-half-inch-long hole in my left thigh from the ejection seat post.

Somehow I tore myself free of the parachute and breast-stroked to the surface. When I got there, the chopper was directly over me. They threw a frogman into the water, and he put a sling on me and they winched me up. However, I couldn't get into the chopper because I couldn't move my legs. So they held me to the side of the chopper and flew me back to the carrier, which took approximately four and a half minutes. It was winter and it was vicious cold.

Once I was back aboard, I remember everything pretty clearly. They took me on a stretcher straight to sick bay and got all my clothes off. Then they might have given me some booze, for all I know.

I had broken every small blood vessel in my legs and couldn't move them for five days. They were swollen giants. It was the impact of the airplane hitting the ocean that did the damage.

I had a choice of being detached from the squadron and going to Tokyo, being treated aboard a Navy hospital ship, or staying with the squadron and being rehabilitated on the ship. I chose the latter. I was concerned that if our squadron was relieved and sent home, or I was detached in Japan, they would reassign me when I got better. Then they might put me in a different squadron and I'd have to start all over again. So by staying with the squadron, when we got relieved, I went home like everybody else.

After five days, they started a rehabilitation program where they used hot packs, cold packs, and had me do minimal exercise until I could do more.

Back then, I was a big, husky guy and weighed 234. But today, I am left with the residue of bad legs. I get a minimal pension for that. I have something called "venous stasis." My legs are almost black and it's because the blood pools down in my legs and doesn't pump back up toward the brain fast enough. I wear stretch stockings the VA gives me.

In retrospect, the Navy would do anything to recover a pilot and to rehabilitate him. Two and a half months after my accident, believe it or not, I was flying again.

Notes
[1]Kimchee is a fermented mixture of cabbage, garlic, and hot peppers.

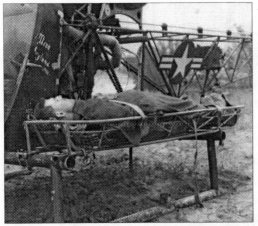

A Marine is about to be evacuated by Bell helicopter. Note the Stokes litter affixed to the skid with pipe clamps. BUMED Archives

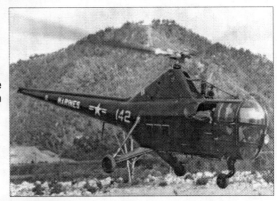

Helicopter picks up a wounded Marine from the battlefield. Note stretcher extending out the open window. BUMED Archives

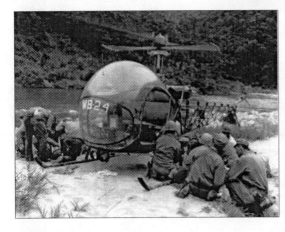

As Marines load a casualty aboard a Bell helicopter, the platoon leader maps the best route to the nearest field hospital. BUMED Archives

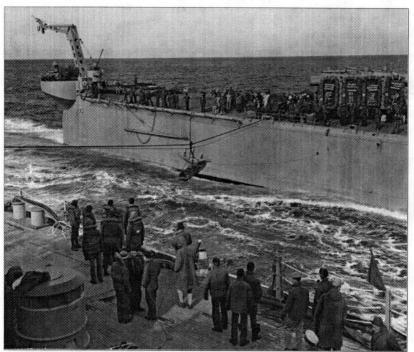

A wounded ROK soldier is transferred by highline from USS *St. Paul* to the 7th Fleet flagship, USS *Wisconsin*. BUMED Archives

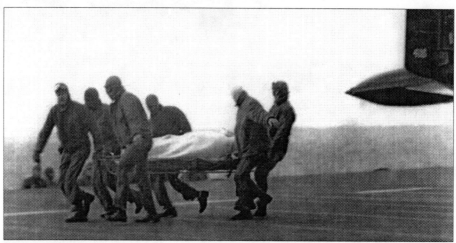

Lt. Cmdr. Aaron Modansky is rushed to sick bay aboard USS *Antietam* following his helicopter rescue. Courtesy of Aaron Modansky

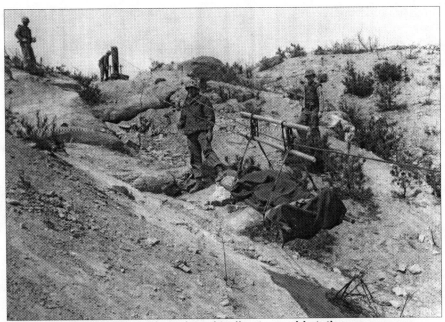

A wounded Marine rides a jury-rigged trolley to an aid station. BUMED Archives

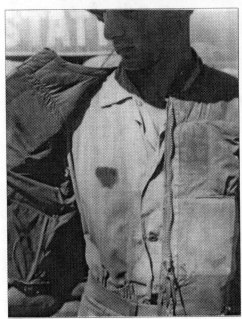

Pfc. Robert Cameron was wearing a flak jacket when he was hit by enemy machine gun fire. The spot shows the size of the bruise caused by a bullet strike. He was treated at a battalion aid station and returned to duty. Eugene Hering Collection, BUMED Archives

Stretchers serve as operating tables at a field hospital. BUMED Archives

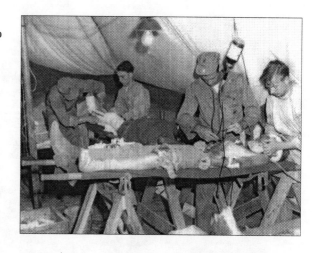

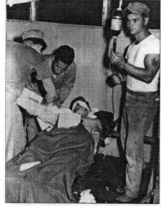

At "Charlie Med," doctors and corpsmen apply a splint to a wounded Marine's arm as he receives a unit of whole blood. BUMED Archives

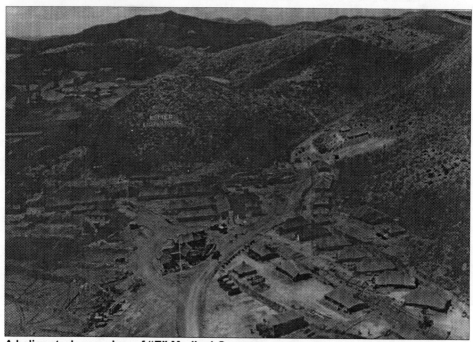

A helicopter's eye view of "E" Medical Company. BUMED Archives

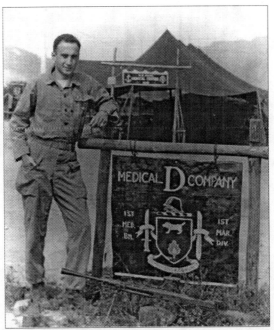

Lt.(j.g.) Hermes Grillo. Courtesy of Hermes Grillo

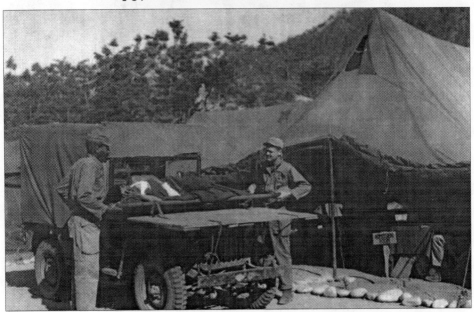

A wounded Marine arrives at a battalion aid station. BUMED Archivesb

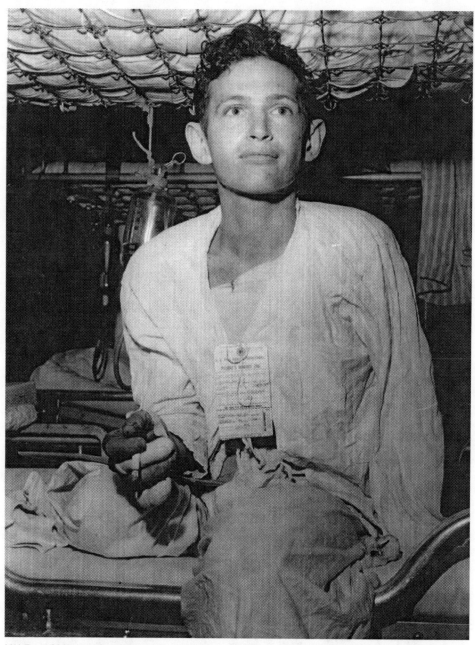

HN Dan Skiles, minus his left arm and right leg, on his way home aboard USS *Haven*. BUMED Archives

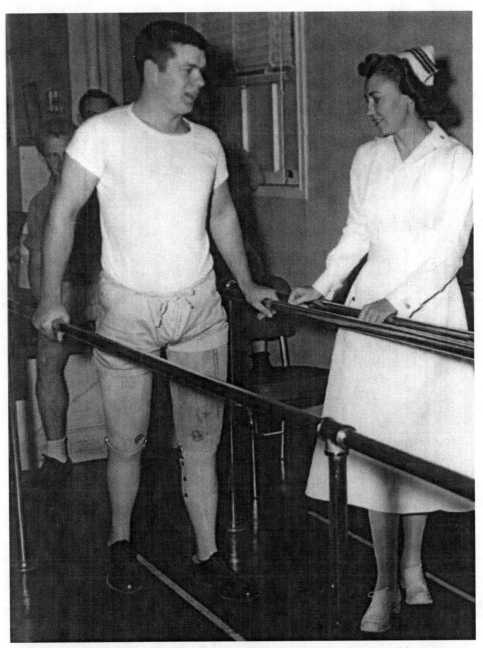

Nurse Lt. Sarah Griffin, herself an amputee, helps a Marine to walk on his new prostheses at Naval Hospital Oakland, California. Naval Historical Center

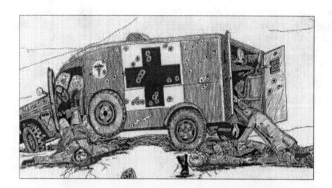

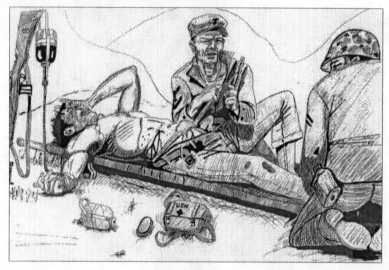

During his recovery, Fenwick drew recollections of his combat experience.
Courtesy of John Fenwick

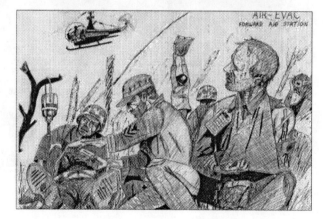

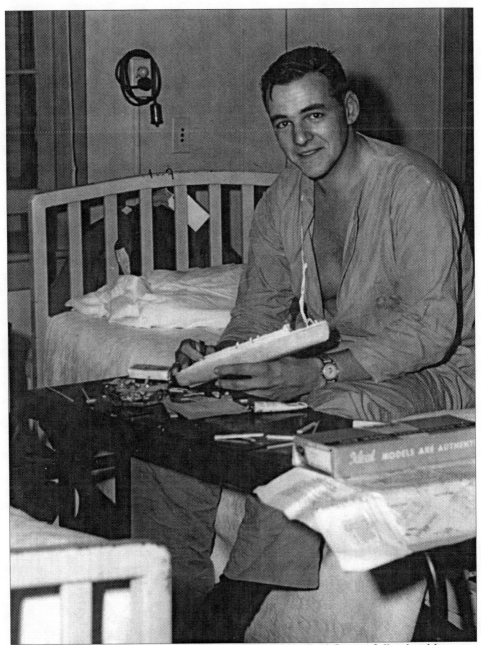

Sgt. John Fenwick recovers at the National Naval Medical Center following his battlefield ordeal. Courtesy of John Fenwick

9

Stalemate

It was January 1951, seven months since the North Korean People's Army had invaded South Korea, triggering a violent and bewildering chain of events. After a very shaky beginning, UN forces routed the invaders and rapidly advanced to the Yalu River, only to be hurled back by hundreds of thousands of communist Chinese soldiers.

Brutal winter fighting occurred throughout the winter, and UN troops withdrew into South Korea with the communists nipping at their heels. Before the situation stabilized, Seoul once more fell into enemy hands. It looked as though the beleaguered nation again teetered on the verge of extinction.

* * *

Surgical Team Eight

Surgical teams were developed to meet the shortage of trained Medical Department personnel in the early phases of the war. They were composed of three medical corps officers and ten corpsmen trained in required field techniques. These teams trained together and were sent to the Far Eastern Theater to serve aboard hospital ships, work at base hospitals in Japan, accompany landing attack parties, and assist medical units of the Marine Corps in the field. At one time there were twenty-five surgical teams. Each team was supposed to have its own equipment and supplies, but training was inadequate and, due to unforeseen circumstances, some missions never came close to success. With UN forces in headlong retreat, Lt.(j.g.) Robert Dobbie of Surgical Team Eight witnessed firsthand the concept's most obvious shortcomings.

The surgical teams were a new concept. There was a surgeon, an anesthesiologist, and a third medical officer who was supposed to be a triage officer. So generally there was a surgeon or a surgical trainee, an internist, and often an ob-gyn man or somebody else who might either help in surgery or give anesthesia. The ten corpsmen with the unit were all first or second class hospital corpsmen and were pretty well trained. Occasionally there was also a chief hospital corpsman.

The concept was that a surgical team could be added to any ship or any shore-based facility and function as an added operating room. And the team carried all its own equipment to function as an operating room. Because of the speed with which we were deployed, we had never trained together; we had never even met each other. The concept was simply a paper concept, and we would have to work things out as time permitted when the opportunity came.

The care of casualties during my TAD [Temporary Additional Duty] at the Yokosuka Naval Hospital on the urology and neurosurgery ward continued through the fall and on into December of 1950. As I had mentioned, in late November and early December, the Chosin frostbite cases descended upon and inundated us until they were able to be evacuated back to either Hawaii or the United States.

The time of the Chinese entry into the war was a terrifying one, and there was a "bug out" retreat down the Korean peninsula. At the time of the Chosin Reservoir and before all the troops were evacuated, there was a plan to parachute the surgical teams into Wonsan, which was the port of debarkation. There we were to help care for wounded Marines who were fighting their way down from the Reservoir. None of us had ever jumped out of a plane, and we were all scared by the prospect when we were put on alert. Nevertheless, we understood the circumstances and were ready to go.

At the last minute, dropping of surgical teams was abandoned in favor of taking them in on PBY seaplanes. But the arrival of the Marines in Wonsan went much better than anticipated. Medical officers were already there, and the evacuation plans for the wounded were such that it seemed more advantageous to evacuate the wounded from Wonsan and take them to Japanese shore-based installations, rather than to send in physicians and surgical teams. So we were spared the seaplane trip or the parachute drop into Wonsan.

On the 30th of December 1950, we were told we would be deployed but not where we were going. We anticipated going to Korea, but at that time there was some thought that the Nationalist Chinese troops from Taiwan might be deployed and we might be sent to Taiwan.

They took us to a warehouse full of all kinds of uniforms and said, "Take whatever you think that you need." Most of us took cold weather gear. I took a jacket and, thinking that might not be enough, I also grabbed a parka. We were also offered sidearms and ammunition. I took both an M1 carbine and a .45 automatic and ammunition for each. Our gear had to be packed into a single duffle bag, and this was the first time we'd seen weapons, helmets, or web belts or bandoliers. None of us really knew how to handle any of these things. Some of the weapons still had their basic Cosmoline grease on them.1 Many of us were unprepared to put on combat gear. Nonetheless, we outfitted ourselves as best we could and cleaned our weapons as best we could, and prepared to leave by plane on New Year's Eve.

We were flown by R4D [DC-3] into Kimpo Airport south of Seoul just when the 8th Army was rapidly retreating down the west coast of Korea. Nobody knew where the pursuing Chinese really were, and Kimpo was in the process of being evacuated as we landed. In fact, we were the last plane in. As soon as they dropped the surgical teams on the tarmac, the plane immediately turned around and took off.

There were all kinds of fires blazing on the periphery of the airport as the troops began to destroy the airport facilities. And we were left alone on the tarmac around all these burning things hopefully waiting for 6 x 6 trucks to come take Surgical Team Eight and the other surgical teams that had come in with us to Inchon.

About eleven o'clock that night the trucks arrived and again we were told we might have to run through roadblocks. We all got in the back of the 6 x 6's and tried to load our weapons. We headed out into the night with great anticipation and some fear.

About an hour later, we arrived at Inchon and were taken to Pier Charlie where an LCM, a small landing craft, ferried us out to the various ships to which we were assigned. Surgical Team Eight was assigned to the USS *Eldorado* [AGC-11]. This was a command ship that looked just like a transport, but was loaded with all kinds of communications and headquarters gear. It was the command ship for amphibious landings, obviously left over from World War II. Just off the port of Inchon, probably a mile or a mile and a half from Pier Charlie, was a fairly large collection of ships. Perhaps one hundred yards away was a hospital ship which was always brightly illuminated. There was also a cruiser with 8-inch guns nearby, maybe a destroyer or two, and two or three or more transports that were busy unloading supplies.

The atmosphere on New Year's Eve was quite tense because a major retreat was under way, and Inchon was being prepared as the port of evacuation for the 8th Army, which was retreating faster than the Chinese could follow.

At this time there were only eight surgical teams, and all eight were deployed either ashore or afloat. One or two of the surgical teams were assigned to the hospital ship; we were assigned to the *Eldorado*. Several surgical teams were assigned to MASH [Mobile Army Surgical Hospital] units because the Army had a great need for surgeons and physicians. In fact, many Navy physicians were required or assigned to work ashore with Army MASH units as individuals. They simply became Army medical officers during their tour in Korea and never saw any shipboard activity at all.

In any event, the line stabilized across the Korean peninsula right about at the 38th Parallel.

* * *

After several months of the bitterest campaigning, the Chinese were expelled from South Korea, and the belligerents faced each other very near the original border between the two Koreas—the 38th Parallel. All across the peninsula—from the Sea of Japan to the Yellow Sea—opposing armies dug in to stay. Even though brief negotiations to stop the conflict began in the summer of 1951 at Kaesong, and later continued in the little truce village of Panmunjom, the war was a stalemate and would remain so for the next two years.

Had a doughboy of 1918 time-traveled to Korea, he would have felt quite at home in the maze of trenches and bunkers that were being constructed along the Main Line of Resistance (MLR). What would have seemed very familiar were the static defense lines, barbed wire, alternating boredom and terror, frequent artillery barrages, individual sniper duels, tasteless rations, vermin, rats, and perpetual filth. On the European Western Front it had been the shelled moonscape of "no-man's-land." Along the MLR it was hand-to-hand fighting for minimal or temporary gain—the Punchbowl, Iron Triangle, Heartbreak Ridge, Bunker Hill, Pork Chop Hill, Chinaman's Hat, Old Baldy, T-Bone, Alligator Jaws, and numbered, rocky, barren hilltops unnamed on any map. Why U.S. forces were in Korea in the first place seemed beyond understanding for most Marines and soldiers contesting this ground. Surviving each day was arduous enough.

Throughout the remainder of 1951 and all of 1952, the bloodletting continued unabated, punctuated by countless skirmishes and battles along the Main Line of Resistance. At Panmunjom, the truce talks dragged on with both sides jockeying for real or perceived strategic advantage. Representatives faced each other day after day, the UN delegates often being subjected to communist insults and ideological diatribes. The pointless meetings frequently adjourned after fits of table-pounding or, more often, after stony silences.

By the spring of 1953, at what became known as the "Nevada Cities," Marines hunkered down in places called Reno, Carson, and Vegas, named, some speculated, for the gambles taken each day in just being there.

* * *

The Bunker War

Hospital corpsman Herbert G. Renner Jr., and his outfit, 2nd Battalion, 5th Marines, occupied positions along the MLR up near "the Parallel." As with most other corpsmen assigned to the Fleet Marine Force, Renner shared their weapons, uniforms, food, and fear. But for the first-aid kit, which he carried behind him to "keep from being identified as a corpsman," he was indistinguishable from the warriors he served. Committing to memory every detail of daily life—and death—Renner remembered forty-eight years later trying to outwit and outlast the wily Chinese enemy he and his comrades commonly referred to as "Gooks" and "Goonies."

In the field in Korea, we corpsmen were outfitted with 782 gear [personal supplies weighing about sixty pounds in full field pack], a .45 automatic pistol model 1911A1 with two extra magazines, holster, and a box of ammo. We also had thermo boots, field boots, and all the other clothing and foul weather gear a Marine had. We carried an M1 rifle with ammo and a bayonet, a Ka-Bar knife, a web belt and all the stuff you can hang on it, but always a canteen containing chlorinated water for washing wounds. Sometimes rifle grenades and launchers could be had.

We never carried any identifying red crosses or serum albumin cans on the helmet as you might see in the movies. We kept grenades in our pockets or hung by a spoon on an outside strap. I never hung them on a strap. We liked concussion grenades for tossing into trenches and bunkers; they weren't as dangerous as fragmentation grenades.

On patrol, a Thompson submachine or a grease gun [submachine gun] was great if you could get one. They both used .45 caliber ammo. The M1 was kept in the bunker and usually only used to defend our static position. Because I was assigned to a fire team and one of my buddies was a BAR man, I carried an extra harness of .30 caliber magazines when we fought on Vegas.

At times we were in blocking positions in that area, especially in March of 1953. … If nothing was going on, about every two weeks we could go back to a field shower unit, bathe, and exchange our clothes for clean ones. If a field mess was found, the cooks would give you some meat, cheese, onions, butter, and bread for sandwiches. They weren't stingy and loaded us up, especially if we had a souvenir to trade.

Everything we ate, with the exception of mess-tent handouts, came in cans called C-rations. Most of the cans contained two things like meat and spaghetti, meat and noodles, ham and lima beans, chicken and vegetables, etc. Another can might have crackers left over from the Civil War, and another had toilet paper, cigarettes, matches, etc. What we didn't like, we dug a hole and buried so a future generation could get a taste of the junk.

The only good thing about being in on an attack or counterattack was the food. We were issued assault rations, little cans of concentrated food and delicious chocolate bars. One I especially liked was the scrambled eggs with ham chunks. When I dreamed, it wasn't about the war. It was about food—steamed crabs and beer, pizza pie—it was just catching on—roasted turkey with all the trimmings, big slabs of baked ham, homemade pies, and ice cream.

Quiet times were used to build up fortifications—sandbagging, digging trenches, bringing up supplies. The wire out front of the MLR had tins cans with stones in them, hung on the wire, and fifty-five-gallon drums of napalm with TNT in the bottom wired to a detonator and dug into the slope at about a forty-five-degree angle.

Minefields were everywhere, especially "bouncing bettys." Going out past the outposts at night you had to step carefully to avoid getting tangled in all the com [communication] wire. I always thought the Gooks had a sure path just to follow the com wire in, if they found it. Com wire was the spaghetti of the battlefield. The paths of our gates were littered with com wire. Patrol after patrol lay down a strand of the twisted black snake. It was slippery even when dry, but it was usually wet and muddy or in the frozen dirt. Twists caught on our boots and became trip wires for people.

We were about to leave a "gate" going on patrol when I had the misfortune of slipping on the carpet of wire and fell off a two-foot-wide path into a coil of concertina wire on my back. I wasn't hurt but was trapped in its clutches. The patrol stopped to salvage their corpsman. I could see their looks of disdain. A hurried call was made explaining the noise of the stones rattling in the cans hung on the wire. What was frightening was the fact that there were mines sown among this wire. I was gingerly extracted and set on my feet again. The patrol leader had a look in his eyes that told me I had come close to getting someone wounded or killed by Marines [attacking] us thinking we were Gooks. Words were never spoken about this episode then or later. I had become the lesson-giver.

Bunkers were built by digging through the side of a deep reverse slope trench at a forty-five-degree angle about three feet wide and about eight feet long, as an entrance way and then, at the end, digging a room about twelve feet by twelve feet. This was all covered with logs, then sandbags up to about three feet thick, then covered with about a foot of earth. A fake chimney was a piece of stovepipe that stopped beneath the earth. The real chimney, for the Yukon stove, came up under the earth, went about twelve feet horizontal, and came out near a bush. This was to prevent the Gooks dropping grenades down our smokestack. The forty-five-degree entrance prevented the enemy shooting in or grenading the bunker. The door was a shelter-half or blanket.

Our bunker was big enough for six of us. It was almost waterproof. Bunks were made of barbed wire stakes laced with com wire to hold the air mattress and mountain sleeping bag. Ammo crates made side tables with a lantern or candle, stools, and a card table. A Yukon stove, similar to a metal box on legs, completed the furnishings, fueled with a jerry can of diesel, a hose, and a drip valve. That stove could get cherry red and damn near run you out of the bunker. When you were on the bunk reading, rats in the overhead logs read along with you and helped themselves to the chow. We had a mutual understanding. Stay off our face when we were sleeping and we wouldn't throw a concussion grenade in the bunker to kill you. I swear to this day that Korean rats could read English and loved our gourmet C-rations. Otherwise, with all the shooting going on, they probably wouldn't have stayed around unless they also enjoyed chewing on a Chinese carcass.

Outside, about twenty feet from the bunker door, was a "piss tube." It was an ammo sleeve of impregnated cardboard stuck in a small soakage pit. It was used instead of going all the way to the head. One night a corpsman from our bunker stepped out to use it just as a mortar round came in, and caught a shell fragment in the buttocks—same as Forrest Gump. An ambulance jeep came up and took him back to a medical battalion. He spent a few weeks sleeping on his belly. He was one of two corpsmen sent to relieve me who got hit before he had spent enough indoctrination time on the MLR to take over on patrols.

On the MLR, we had a .50-caliber machine gun mounted in a covered firing position, and the gunner was very good at snapping off one round when the situation called for it. With nothing much to do, I just happened to be at the firing position while he was watching a Gook through a telescopic sight, which was mounted on the gun. The Gook was digging in a trench. He would go down in the trench, get a basket of dirt, come up a ladder, and throw the dirt over the edge of the trench. The gunner told me to take a pair of binoculars he had and watch the Gook the next time he came up the ladder. He came up again and a .50-caliber slug hit him and threw him on the back of the trench. The gunner said he had been tweaking the gun in on the Gook for the last ten minutes or so.

The worst weapon of war, in my opinion, was napalm. We were on patrol at night and came across a group of Gooks who had been hit with the stuff. They were fried in grotesque positions, some sitting, some kneeling, and some on their faces in the dirt. Some were still holding their weapons. The smell of burned flesh still lingered. Should you want to remember the smell of a battlefield, just smell the opening of a cartridge case that has recently been fired. That's the smell that permeates the haze.

Marines who had been in close combat for a while could tell you the type of ordnance being flung at us by the sound of the shell in the air, or by the explosion, or both. I could determine the small stuff. Burp guns sounded like "burps." A single "crack" was a rifle bullet. Multiple cracks and a lot of dirt thrown up was a machine gun. I had a hard time telling apart fragmentation grenades and 60mm mortars.

One day I was helping Bill Sterns, a radioman, string some com wire along the trench. He got up on the edge to put some dirt over the wire to hold it down when "crack," a bullet snapped right by his head. I wasn't more than a couple of feet from him and heard the sound like a whip crack. Needless to say, we kept our heads down and tried to spot the sniper to no avail.

Artillery shells and mortar rounds that the Chinese shot at us were called "incoming" and the shells going toward them were called "outgoing." The incoming had an eerie whistle. The outgoing big shells chugged like a train on a hill.

Mortar crews had a pit lined around the sides with sandbags and a small shelf where they planted aiming stakes. Depending on the distance the projectile was to be fired, they put increments on the fins to give the shot a boost.

When I was new on the line, the Marines would tell me what incoming had just hit in our area. Mines made all sorts of different noises, depending upon their size and the depth they were buried. A 90mm tank gun muzzle blast got your attention. A bazooka was one of those whizz-bangs that threw up smoke and dust. I remember when a Gook 82mm mortar found our "four-holer" head. No one was in it at the time, but it certainly made a mess—turds and slime everywhere. It took hours to find it all and cover it with dirt. Field sanitation went to hell that day.

The searchlight at Panmunjom stayed on all night and pointed straight up so no one would shell or bomb them. We used to think of stealing the light and bringing it over to our hill so we wouldn't get shelled or bombed.[2] A map I saw indicated we were on Hill 126. Three enemy hills were in front of us—Betty Grable—because it had a long leg, Hill 98, and another hill that went by Frisco or Garry. They were napalmed, bombed, and rocketed by our airplanes quite often.

Going back to the showers and getting clean clothes could be dangerous. A plane bombed us once, and we had to jump into a rice paddy to get cover behind a retaining wall. A piece of shell fragment, larger than my hand and as thick, slid in the mud right in front of my eyes, turning iridescent colors as it cooled.

When not working on fortifications, we could write letters, cook some chow, wash clothes or ourselves, or clean a weapon. Some nights, when not on patrol, we were assigned duty on the sound-powered phones, logging the watches and outposts checking in. That was a welcome change—with hot coffee all night.

Worm pills and DDT powder had to be distributed when the lice and worms started to itch. You could tell when someone was bothered with them because you saw him scratching his head, his butt, or both. They said malaria and hemorrhagic fevers were present in Korea, but I never saw a case.

Unless something was going on, we slept during the day and patrolled at night. Patrols were called Cadillacs, Chevrolets, Buicks, and some other names. I can't remember which were which, but they were combat, ambush, recon, etc., patrols. I liked the ambush patrol in the spring because we could lie out under the stars and wait for the Gooks to find us, which they seldom did. In winter, the recon patrols were the best. You could keep warm moving around. Combat patrols involved getting into the Gooks' trenches and blowing up their outpost bunkers. These weren't fun because the Gooks would get mad as hell and shoot back, or you had to break your butt getting away from a satchel charge blast.

Moonlit nights were doubly dangerous for obvious reasons. Sometimes we didn't have to go out very far. If it was too bright, we'd just hang around an outpost or stay close in. No sense getting slaughtered by the Gook mortars. The story was that every Gook had a mortar and a hundred ammo carriers. They were good shots! Every now and then, we would find a couple of their lookouts in a shell hole not far from our lines and usually half frozen in the winter. The "G-men" liked to get them for questioning before they were sent back to a prisoner compound. Our company commander dearly loved prisoners. I think he got a bonus for every Gook captured.

Small patrols were led by a sergeant or better, and platoon size by an officer. The larger the number on patrol the more the danger. I could never hear very well, but it seemed to me I could hear every footstep of everyone around me. The patrol leader usually put me one man forward of the tail gunner. Because we had good leaders, we took very few casualties and none of them serious on the patrols I accompanied—and I went on a lot of them. We took more casualties in blocking actions from incoming artillery.

About an hour or two after nightfall, the Marines assembled behind the MLR for the night's patrol. There was no inspection by the officer or NCO who would lead the patrol. There was no need. The Marines came clothed, equipped, and ready for the job ahead. Rounds were chambered, weapons checked on "safe." The type of patrol was discussed, again detailing the orders given earlier in the day. Last-minute questions were answered, the men were assigned their positions, and the patrol headed for the MLR and the zigzag trench that descended the forward slope. This all took about ten minutes.

Canteens were full so they wouldn't slosh and we wouldn't drink again until heading back many hours later. Food was carried unwrapped—usually some candy. We would have had our final meal for the day and our bladders and bowels were emptied. The patrol might last five hours or more. Of course, we never smoked or talked. The muffled sound of the patrol leader's voice on the phones or radio might be heard if you were near enough. There were no incoming calls on the radio—at least, I never heard one.

The trench was deep, about head high, as we descended. As we passed the machine gun bunker that protected the "gate," com wire from a spool on a man's back was connected for the sound-powered phones and the announcement made that the patrol was departing. The trench ended and became a shallow gully as we stepped into no-man's-land single file. Fourteen men would be strung out almost 175 feet from the far point to tail gunner. We might be anywhere from 500 to 1,500 yards from our designated point of action, regardless of whether it was an ambush, recon, or combat patrol. By this time our eyes were fully acclimated to the dark, a process that took about forty-five minutes.

Assuming we were on a combat patrol to engage the enemy on his home turf, we headed for his lines in a direction that earlier patrols hadn't taken recently to avoid being ambushed. As we approached the enemy hills, the crests were outlined in the skylight. This was especially true if the night was crisp and clear with no high clouds to obstruct the starlight. To the enemy looking down in our direction, he would see nothing but blackness.

Off in the distance, to the east or west, there might be a fire fight or an artillery mission being fired, and the sound rumbled down the valleys. Sometimes the pinpoints of flashes could be seen near the crest of a hill—maybe ours, maybe theirs. Rocket ripples were an amazing thing to watch—unless you happened to be the recipient. Way out of our sector a tank searchlight illuminated the battlefield as the enemy probed someone else's section of the MLR. The shaft of light was too far away to make shadows follow our footsteps.

As we neared their hills, our patrol leader looked for their paths through the minefields. If they were home and heard us, they would hurl grenades down from their positions. We would withdraw to a safe location, and the leader would call down a mission on their heads. If they didn't suspect our approach, they were doomed. Our grenades and small arms fire would make short work of the operation. Many times neither happened; they weren't home. We could slide into their trenches, look around, and rest a bit. Further objectives weren't usually considered that night because other Marine patrols were out doing their thing, and we didn't need to run into them. Regardless of the outcome, we had to get back to our lines well before daylight or the Gooks would have us for breakfast. To this day, I dislike being out at night in unlit places.

One night we got trapped in a small bowl with low ridges on both sides and the front. The Gooks were on the other side of the front ridge and must have thought we had crossed it and were heading for them. They were pounding the area with small 61mm mortars and spraying it with machine gun fire. We were in platoon strength. The lieutenant called in machine gun fire just over our heads toward the front ridge, and had a mortar barrage box us in on three sides so we could escape from the rear of the bowl. Our machine gunners fired so low that a man with a spool of com wire on his back, who was trapped near the top of the front ridge, got some rounds through the spool. We got out of the bowl and tried to flank the Gooks, but they were wise to us and started to walk mortars toward us. The patrol was aborted and we went back to the MLR. There were no casualties that night.

Somewhere near the Nevada Cities we got smashed by what someone said was our own artillery—105mm. I never found out for sure. I guess I really didn't want to know. We lost about a dozen Marines, some killed. The "chiggy bearers" came up to take out the bodies and the non-walking wounded. Those were brave, little old guys from South Korean labor battalions. They were tough little devils who were too old or too young to be in fighting units. They'd come up with litters and take the wounded out.[3]

I had heard the shells exploding as they came toward us up the gully we were in, and got up under a washed-out tree root beside a dry stream bed. I pulled my helmet down so hard it probably covered my feet. The blast of a shell hitting above me bounced me around, covered me with debris from the tree roots, and I couldn't hear for a while.

Artillerymen considered themselves the "kings of the battlefield" because their massed fire could cause such destruction. The steel rain from their guns could destroy the fighting ability of whole companies of Chinese. If they were kings, the mud Marines were the "knights" who met the enemy in the field in close combat.

Another time, we were positioned in a field below some of our tanks that were sitting on a ridge. We were resting and eating what we had gotten from a field mess on a reverse slope near the front. I guess the Gooks saw the tanks and started shooting at them. The short rounds fell on us. It was broad daylight. Huge pieces of shell fragments got some of the guys. I finally got to a guy who had caught one in the head. It took off most of the right side. I put an abdominal battle dressing over the wound, more to hide it, and gave him a shot of morphine. Neither, of course, did any good. I just stayed with him until he expired. I didn't recognize him because of the size of the wound, and I long ago forgot the name on his dog tag.

During the Nevada Cities battles, we were called up from reserve to be thrown into a blocking action and later into an attack on Vegas. A few things happened that are vivid to this day. We were passing an aid station; slightly wounded and dead were outside. I went in to look for some replacement medical supplies. I never got much. Medical officers and corpsmen were working on the seriously wounded. The stench, gore, and foul air in that dark bunker with the cries and groans of the wounded were just too much to bear. I had to get out into the fresh air and see what I could do for those outside.

Another vivid memory was a run along a rice paddy wall when a 76mm opened up on us. A Marine far in front jumped into a shell hole for cover. A shell fell right into the same hole with him. There was little left. I continued to run toward the end of the wall for cover when I heard a round whiz by. I fell, and sticking up from the dirt were the three prongs of a "bouncing betty" antipersonnel mine. After I got up and ran into a shallow ravine, there was a Marine who had had an emotional breakdown being sent back to the rear. He was the first and last one I ever saw.

Sometime during the fight I remember the word being passed that Major Lee and Captain Walz were killed. We were headed up a lower slope of Vegas when an enemy mortar barrage came in. I had flopped down beside a radioman who had one of those big radios with the long whip antenna. He may have been a forward observer. When the barrage lifted, I got up to run and the radioman didn't move. I checked him out and discovered something had gone through his helmet and destroyed the top of his head.

There weren't many wounded because there weren't many of us left. I still remember the eyes of the dead Marines. They were open and seemed to be staring blankly into the haze of the battlefield. Those whose eyes were closed appeared to be asleep. The bodies of the recent dead, who hadn't yet been moved and covered, were sometimes in the strangest positions and were probably running when they caught a shell fragment.

During an attack on an enemy position, you started out with the whole unit all around you. Then you stopped to treat a wounded man and looked around, noting that there were few, if anyone, around. It was a stop-and-catch-up situation. I had a tendency to get disoriented except for the fact that the usual direction was "up" the hill. I never had a map or compass. When I got lost, usually a Marine came along who knew the proper direction.

We spent the night fitfully sleeping in trenches that were no more than two feet deep, having been blown in by artillery and mortar fire. One morning, very early, before the morning mist had cleared, we were attacked by the Chinese. Leo Kelly had his BAR working and was cutting them down as they came out of the mist and smoke. They were too far away to see their features. They fell like rag dolls. I was carrying ammo for him and squatted beside him and handed him magazines when he ran out of his supply. The Gooks left and the remainder of the day was without much disturbance.

When we were relieved, I carried a bazooka tube back down the hill. The hill was littered with personal weapons, both ours and the Chinese. We broke what we couldn't carry in case the Chinese were to overrun the hill again. I can't remember what the weather was like except there was mud. Maybe it was clear above the battlefield haze which could obscure the sky, or there could have been low clouds scudding over. There had been full moons that could be seen sometimes at night. A moon's light shone through the clouds and haze. I don't remember going back to the MLR or anything else after leaving that hill. It seems to be a blank.

The battles of the Nevada Cities had raged for five days [26 to 30 March 1953]. Vegas remained ours; Reno was lost forever. Carson was never completely overrun to my knowledge, or, if it was, it was immediately retaken. Many years later I learned that Carson was lost that April when it was in the hands of the Army.

I was six feet two inches and about 190 pounds when I arrived at Camp Pendleton. When I boarded the troopship going home from the "Land of the Morning Calm," I weighed about 165 pounds.

* * *

One of the most important lifesaving innovations of the Korean War was body armor. Although the "flak vest" had been developed by Navy and Army laboratories during World War II, weight and design flaws precluded its widespread use. The end of hostilities saw a lapse in body armor research and development.

The Korean War revived the quest for effective armor that would protect the wearer's chest, abdomen, and back. The guts of the vest consisted of a fiberglass laminate—Doron—that had been bonded at high temperature and formed into curved plates that were sewn inside the nylon vest. Although the armor could not prevent penetration by high-velocity rifle or machine gun bullets, tests showed that it could stop .45 caliber bullets fired either from an automatic pistol at close range or from a submachine gun at a distance of fifteen feet. It could also stop most hand grenade fragments.

In early 1951, a joint Army-Navy mission began testing forty sets of prototype jackets fabricated by the Naval Medical Research Laboratory. The flak vests were then sent to Korea to be distributed among personnel in one Marine and two Army regiments. Lt. Cmdr. Frederick Lewis, a Navy physician, designed the armor with the assistance of another Navy doctor, Cmdr. John Cowan. Both physicians went to Korea to monitor the trials, code-named "Operation Boar." During the two-month test period, six thousand soldiers and Marines wore the vests.

The prototypes were heavy and uncomfortable in the hot Korean summer. Some troops discarded the vests. Others found it difficult to shoulder their weapons because the plates rode up and became cumbersome. Nevertheless, the flak vests began saving lives immediately. Their use decreased chest wounds by 60 percent. Men hit by shell and mortar fragments and by 7.62mm burp gun slugs walked away with bruises rather than mortal wounds.

Taking the troops' criticism to heart, the Naval Medical Field Research Laboratory at Camp Lejeune, North Carolina, modified the vest. The improved M-1952 flak vest weighed 7¾ pounds and contained overlapping Doron plates which covered the lower chest, back, and abdomen. Another type of armor, made of a flexible, woven nylon, covered the upper chest and shoulders. This improved vest became so popular that few soldiers or Marines would go in harm's way without it.

* * *

James Sartorelli was a corporal attached to a weapons company, 2nd Battalion, 1st Marines, when he was hit. His flak jacket literally made the difference between life and death.

We were issued flak vests when we got up on the line in June of '52. They looked like a big vest and they came down to your waist. They had hard sections built in to protect your chest and back. Being in a weapons company, we used to catch a lot of flak. When the enemy knew we were coming, they called in everything on us—artillery, mortars, plus rifle and automatic weapons fire.

On 23 August 1952, about one o'clock in the morning, we were sent out to reinforce Fox Company in holding Bunker Hill for three days. The weather was extremely foggy. It was so foggy, in fact, that we had to hang on to each other's shirttails. We were loaded down with our heavy and light machine guns, flame throwers, rockets, and ammunition. They told us not to talk or make a sound.

Suddenly the sergeant in front of me stopped. I didn't see him so I ran into him. When I stopped, the guy behind me did the same thing and ran into me. We all went over the edge of a ravine and the whole damn mess of us landed one on top of the other. The sergeant and I were on the bottom of the pile. I was carrying a pack of rocket ammunition on my back at the time, and my assistant had the flame thrower and tank. I thought my back had been broken.

Because it had been raining steadily, we lay there in six inches of water. Every time I tried to get my head above the water, someone else would topple over the edge of the ravine, land on me, and push my head under. The only one who wasn't hurt was our corpsman.

I began swearing and hollering from the pain and the corpsman kept telling me to quiet down because there were Gooks around. But I was in so much pain, I told him to let them come. I'd rather get shot than bear the pain I had in my back. I couldn't even sling my rifle after that. I had to hold it the way you might carry a dinner pail. We were in the ravine for a half hour to an hour before a scout came and led us to Bunker Hill.

On 23 and 24 August, there was no action because it was too foggy and rainy so, in our area, a bunker was built and foxholes were sandbagged.

On the 25th it cleared off and one of our men stood up to stretch and that was it. He was shot and killed immediately. I can't even remember his name. When you were over there, you didn't have buddies; they didn't last long. I was assigned to a machine gun bunker but was called back. Our sergeant, who landed in the ravine with us, was sent back to the MLR because his injured leg was giving him problems. So I was put in the sergeant's place in charge of our squad.

As it got dark, we started getting incoming artillery, mortars, and enemy fire. I was in a two-man foxhole with a BAR [Browning Automatic Rifle] man and there were four or five men spread out in one-man foxholes. Off to the right was a light machine gun bunker which I found out later got a direct hit by an artillery shell. Two were killed in that foxhole and one got a concussion. That's when the Gooks started attacking our line.

On the left, we had another foxhole position with a light machine gun in it. When they opened up firing, they drew enemy fire and we fired back. While the machine gun was firing, the Gooks threw in concussion hand grenades to knock it out. At that time, flares were going up and I saw a hand grenade roll down the gunner's back as he ducked and held on to the machine gun. The grenade blew him and his partner out of the hole. I thought they were both killed, but a few minutes later they were packing up their machine gun and moving up to a foxhole closer to the enemy. I later heard that it was a lieutenant who was in the foxhole with him. The flak jackets they wore saved them.

I soon ran out of ammo, so I went back to our ammo bunker to replenish my supply. But we had caught so much incoming from the enemy and even our own artillery that our ammo bunker had been blown up. So I was forced to pick up ammunition scattered on the ground. I was looking for clips for my M1 but could only pick up so much, and then I had to get back to my foxhole.

As I was going back up the hill, the enemy began throwing hand grenades over. You could see them flipping through the air with sparks coming from the handles. They were like those German potato masher grenades with the wooden handles. They overthrew us with most of them because they were easier to throw than our grenades.

They couldn't have been more than twenty feet from us. Usually they had one guy who carried them in a pack on his back, and another guy would throw them. They worked as a team. Anyway, I dove for my foxhole but a grenade had gotten there ahead of me, and I landed right on top of it. It exploded against my chest and blew me right back out where I started from. My flak jacket was all torn to pieces. These were concussion rather than fragmentation grenades, otherwise I wouldn't have survived.

Nevertheless, a fragment hit me in the throat. As I lay in the cold mud, I could feel my hand get warm. I reached around my throat and found a hole. I stuck my finger in it to stop the bleeding. I cursed awhile figuring that I had had it. Then I yelled for a corpsman and someone called back and said, "If you can swear that much, your throat can't be that bad."

I then went back to a bunker which had been turned into an aid station. It was loaded with wounded. The only way I could get fixed was to stick just my head in the door. A corpsman looked at the wound in my neck, bandaged it, and told me not to move my head because the fragment was against my jugular vein. He was afraid it would cut it and I would bleed to death. He told me to watch another Marine in a bunker nearby who had a concussion and needed to be watched so he wouldn't be wandering around.

The battle was still going on. I got hit around 11:00 P.M. and we got off the hill the next morning, 26 August, just as it was getting light. Five from our group who were wounded were able to help each other back to the MLR. Because of the land mines, I helped the guy with the concussion to stay on the path.

The real badly wounded were flown out to a field hospital. The rest of us, who didn't look too bad, were taken off the line in amtracs to a field hospital. The doctors there didn't know whether to take the fragment out of my throat or leave it in because it was right next to the jugular. But they figured that if they sent me back, my neck might move and the jugular would be severed. So finally they took it out right there. I was put on the hospital ship USS *Repose* and later flown to Naval Hospital Yokosuka, Japan. I was twenty-three, the old man of the bunch.

I figure it was that flak vest that saved my life otherwise that grenade would have finished me off. When we were attacked, we would call in an air burst and catch the Gooks out in the open. The flak jackets protected us from most of the shrapnel although there were some who were wounded or killed by it.

Notes

[1] A heavy grease used to protect weapons from the elements.

[2] The searchlight also was a warning for aircraft to keep their distance.

[3] These Korean laborers were originally designated the Civil Transportation Corps, and later the Korean Service Corps. They carried supplies strapped to A-frame packs (*Chigae*).

10

Surgeons at the Front

*T*he 1st Provisional Marine Brigade first set out for Korea in the summer of 1950. The hastily organized 1st Medical Battalion, which provided medical support first for the Brigade and then the 1st Marine Division, consisted of a hospital and service (H&S) company, two hospital companies (A and B), and three collecting and clearing companies (C, D and E). Clearing platoons of Companies C, D, and E operated field hospitals, and the collecting platoons supported infantry battalions. This was the configuration that supported the successful Inchon invasion that September.

A year later, with the war bogged down in stalemate, many small and large unit actions, accompanied by punishing artillery duels, were generating casualties at a horrific rate. To take care of their own, the Army had well equipped Mobile Army Surgical Hospitals (MASHs) staffed with experienced surgeons and nurses. The Marines, as always, depended on the Navy Medical Department.

As the character of the war had changed in its first year, so had medical facilities and their organization. Operating in tents within four miles of the fighting, the 1st Marine Division relied upon "Charlie" Med, "Dog" Med, and "Easy" Med hospital companies. These were small, spartan, definitive-care surgical hospitals that were often capable of performing miracles with inadequate personnel and equipment. Able Med, farther from the front, had become the specialty and holding company, and Baker Med was left with the Division rear echelon far south in Masan and out of the picture. Staffing these meager facilities were the too-few experienced career Navy surgeons and the not-so-plentiful Reserve "jaygees," some just days from stateside hospital residencies.

* * *
"Don't Let Me Die!"
Howard Sirak was a graduate of Ohio State Medical School, and, as with the many other young physicians who were called up for Korea, he had gotten his education under the V-12 program. "I had an opportunity to do research at NIH [National Institutes of Health], but I didn't want to pull any strings. And so I went," he recalls. "I didn't mind it, but I did mind leaving my family and young baby daughter. It nearly broke my heart."

By Christmas 1950, Sirak was in Korea where his surgical skills were soon put to use. The military situation had continued to deteriorate as the Chinese moved toward the 38th Parallel, and UN troops staggered back into South Korea before the onslaught.

We landed at Kimpo. The buildings were all shell- and bullet-pocked. I remember it was a cold, snowy, winter night and we were all heavily clothed. The natives, the poor devils, were on the roads moving back [south]. They were in sandals with feet bare. It was a very cold night. I thought they had a remarkable resistance to the cold and admired their resilience.

Korea was a very primitive country at the time. Our military was worried that the Chinese might swing to the coast, cut the troops off, pinning them against the coast at Inchon. There were tremendous tides there, and that would have made evacuation difficult. They put us on ships at Inchon, but didn't know exactly how they were going to use us at the time.

After the Chosin retreat, the evacuees flooded the Naval hospital at Yokosuka, where I was at the time. I had never seen so many cases of gangrenous black feet, noses, and extremities. The arterioles are small, muscular walled vessels—the tiny ones—that are precapillary. And the cold, of course, would cause them to contract. The red cells would clump inside them so that the tissue beyond, unable to receive nourishment, would die and become gangrenous.

There was not a lot you could do for the gangrene. We waited for there to be a clear demarcation between the pink skin and necrotic tissue. The dead tissue became black as coal. Then it was easy to distinguish what was dead and what was vital. We had people coming over from the States who experimented with cortisone to see if it would increase the circulation or diminish the amount of tissue lost. But that didn't work. At one time we had over five thousand frostbite cases in the hospital.

It was already 1951 when I was assigned to Easy Med. It was located pretty far north along the Soyanggang River, and was the farthest north definitive medical unit. We got the casualties right off the field, right after the corpsmen in the forward aid stations gave them plasma, and stopped the bleeding so that they could evacuate them to us. There was a tiny airstrip adjacent to our camp, where helicopters and sometimes P-51s landed. The casualties would pour in, brought by DUKWs [amphibious trucks], helicopters with stretchers on the skids on each side, or by ambulances.

There were sleeping, supply, and storage tents at Easy Med, but the unit was kept small so that it could be very mobile. We had tents with what I used to call "wall-to-wall carpeting" because it was all a rice paddy that had been bulldozed flat. We had an operating room tent and a triage tent attached to it. This triage area was where the casualties were first brought to be assessed, transfused, and have their bloody clothing removed and searched for explosives. The clothing was then thrown into a bonfire. Once, a grenade [from someone's pocket] was overlooked. There was quite an explosion and we could hear the shrapnel whistling over our heads. Luckily, no one was injured.

When we first went over to Korea we took a lot of gear in a box as big as a coffin. I don't know how many hundred pounds it weighed. Unfortunately, when we opened it, it was filled with equipment, none of which we could use. There was stuff as outdated as Mercurochrome. Who in 1950 remembered using Mercurochrome? Well, I remembered it because I was born in the '20s and my mother used to dab some on my scratches. By 1950, it was a totally obsolete drug. The box also had components that had to be hand-mixed to make a plaster cast, and drip ether and masks that dated to World War I! Well, you can't operate on young men with equipment that was so obsolete. We were so angry and disappointed that we had been supplied with junk that we took all this useless material and threw it into a rice paddy.

When the Marines were on the assault, we would be swamped with wounded. The normal sequence at Easy Med was like this. We first had to decide whether a given wounded was salvageable. We had to direct our efforts to those who could be saved so we had to make decisions about who would go into the operating tent in what order of priority.

Once they were triaged, the patients were transfused, examined, and cleaned up as best we could. They would come into the O.R. and we would just go to work. One time my team and I operated thirty-two straight hours without eating or sleeping because the patient load was so enormous.

The nights and days seemed to blend imperceptibly.

We had a good anesthesiologist whom I talked into coming over from the Yokosuka Naval Hospital. You needed a really good anesthesiologist and good anesthesia equipment. Someone finally helped us get a good machine. We could put these kids to sleep safely and still get good relaxation of the abdominal muscles. I think we may have used a little pentothal for induction, but not to carry the patient during the procedure. You don't get enough abdominal muscular relaxation with pentothal. And if you give too much, then you have postoperative problems. I can't remember what inhalational anesthesia we used, but it would have been one of the commonly used inhalational types.

We had suction. We had good lights. Because they hadn't been supplied to us, we had malleable retractors made by the men in the nearby engineering camp who split some copper tubing longitudinally and flattened it.

We didn't have any x-ray equipment up there, and that made things pretty complicated for locating fragments. But the main thing was to solve the problems with the holes or tears in the gut, or in the chest, and to control bleeding. You had to be very careful not to overlook a small perforation in the gut or a laceration of a major blood vessel. You might get only one crack at that patient. If feces continued to spill into the peritoneal cavity, the patient would likely die or have serious complications. It was necessary for us to "run" the bowel from one end to the other and check all the organs and retroperitoneal area.

We didn't experiment with vascular surgery at all, but repaired arterial tears if they were repairable. If somebody had a lacerated carotid I could repair it. We didn't have [artificial] grafts in those days, and they probably would not have been suitable because you had to deal with dirty wounds—contaminated wounds. If you used a foreign body (a prosthetic graft), your chances of success would be small.

For suturing we used catgut, which is an absorbable suture. We worried about using a foreign body in a contaminated area. Remember, you had no time preoperatively to use intestinal antibiotics to reduce the bacterial flora like you would if you were doing an elective procedure on a patient here in the States. You always had to be concerned about infection. Silk, of course, is a foreign body, so we didn't use any except for vascular repairs. If the patient developed an abscess, we would have to re-operate and that would have increased the risk. Laparoscopy didn't exist.

For antibiotics, we had chloramphenicol, which was later eliminated because of its toxic effect on bone marrow. We also had sulfas, streptomycin, terramycin, and penicillin.

While I was at Easy Med, I saw more dirty bellies than I care to see again. Usually there were cinders, gravel, grass, clothing, and other foreign material that would be blown into and through the abdominal wall. This made the skin a difficult surface to render sterile.

I really haven't thought very much about all this in the last fifty years. I think it's one of those things that the mind purposely blanks out. When you carry a youngster into an operating tent [who is]screaming, "Don't let me die! Don't let me die," it makes an indelible impression on you.

* * *

Mini-MASH

Howard Browne had been in love with the Navy since an aunt gave him a "Dixie Cup" sailor hat in 1935. During World War II, while attending the University of Oklahoma, he enlisted in the Navy Reserve V-1 program. After finishing their freshman year, the V-1 students suddenly were converted to V-12 cadets and ordered to active duty. "We learned the rudiments: how to salute, dress and march and how to make an inadequate issue of two white uniforms stretch by wearing one and washing the other every night." The war ended before he graduated, and

Browne continued his pre-med education before attending Northwestern University Medical School.

Halfway through his internship, as with other graduates who had attended medical school on the government's dime, Browne received the famous "Forrestal suasion telegram."[1] Paraphrased, the telegram read, "Since the Navy paid for part of your education and is short of doctors on active duty, we consider that you have a moral, if not a legal, obligation to volunteer for active duty after you finish your internship. If you will volunteer for one year of active duty, the Navy will give you the pay and allowances of a lieutenant, junior grade, during your internship."

It was 1949 and Browne and several of his friends "beat it down to the recruiting office and signed up." When his internship ended, he received orders to Naval Hospital Bremerton, Washington. In 1951, he finally had the opportunity to get World War II off his back. "When news came of the horrible trap at the Chosin Reservoir the Marines had fought their way out of, I just had to volunteer for the FMF [Fleet Marine Force]." Dr. Browne was soon on his way to the front.

I off-loaded at Pusan and flew to an airstrip where a Marine 6 x 6 International truck was waiting to transport me. I sat up front with the driver, looking apprehensively out the window. I didn't know that Division was a safe distance behind the lines. At one point, the driver opened the glove compartment, reached in, pulled out a .45 and laid it on the seat between us. "What's that for?" I said.

"Ambush. Last week a buddy of mine got ambushed by NK [North Korean] guerrillas about here."

The terrorization was complete when I stepped out of the truck at Division and saw a dead corpsman lying on the ground awaiting disposition.

The next day I was driven to Headquarters 3rd Battalion, 11th Marines, an artillery battalion. We stopped at the sick bay tent and I met the man I was relieving, Lt.(j.g.) Robert Shoemaker, and my corpsmen. I have never been treated so well in my life. Shoemaker made sure I wore my helmet at all times and had a deep foxhole ready for me. He didn't want anything to happen to me before he left for home the next day.

I have to say that other than being scared all the time, I wasn't a bit worried. I could be hit by enemy mortars or artillery, attacked by infiltrators, or step on or drive over a mine, but I knew the Marines wouldn't leave me behind. I knew from a classmate and one or two other doctors that the Army had bugged out and left them and their aid stations behind. I don't know what the casualty rate of Army doctors was, but the Marines lost only one, Lt.(j.g.) Peter Arioli, shot by a sniper at the Reservoir.[2]

My duties were simple. We tried to hold regular morning and evening sick call, but our tent flap was open at all times. When we had casualties, we'd give them first aid and evacuate them to the closest medical company. A day or so after I arrived, the Battalion exec, Maj. Norman "Red" Miller, took me on rounds of the position. In each tent he'd open the lid of the jerry can and sniff. I thought, "How nice. He's making sure the boys aren't keeping water in gasoline cans."

One night shortly after, someone scratched at the flap of my tent. I opened it and a man said, "Hey, Doc, come over to the Com tent—and bring your canteen cup."

The communication guys had just opened a jerry can of raisin jack and were reduced to slurred speech and giggles. One explained, "This batch went five days. We call that 'VO [Very Old].' Sometimes we let it go seven. That's 'VVO [Very, Very Old].'"

From this I learned that the surgeon, who got a ration of ethyl alcohol for medical use and a few little bottles of LeJon brandy for resuscitation, was second in popularity only to the cook, who could supply sugar, yeast, and canned fruit cocktail—the ingredients of raisin jack.

Korea was not fought under the Geneva Convention, so we didn't wear Red Cross armbands. If our hospital tents were identified, it was only to keep our own planes from bombing us. Medics had to carry a weapon. To enforce the discipline, we couldn't get in the chow line without wearing our weapon. Mine was an M1 carbine, a real pain to be tied to. So the idea was to get in good with the battalion armorer. A little sick bay alcohol got me a swap of the carbine for a .45, which was much easier to carry.

In June–July [1951], the Division was on the rebound and we moved fairly often. Each position we set up in had been occupied by the enemy and he had coordinates of every site. He knew where we'd put the guns, the Fire Direction Center, etc. The first time I came under fire we had 90mm mortars ranged on us. I hid in a bunker, scared out of my wits. Two Marines were calmly arguing whether boot camp at San Diego was as tough as at Parris Island. I figured if those guys weren't scared, why should I be? And I was comforted if not relieved. Then came the call "Corpsman!" which I also responded to. A mortar bomb had landed close to a tent and a couple of boys were hit. One was screaming frantically, clutching his groin, which was very bloody. "The bastards have castrated me, Doc!" voicing the soldier's worst fear.

I pried his hands away and the corpsman held them as I cut away his utilities. I tried to reassure him with something like, "You won't have to join the choir; it's a clean hit through your foreskin." I evacuated him where the surgeon probably completed the circumcision.

In the summer of '51, we were moving forward very fast. The Punchbowl, the Hwachon Reservoir, and Taegu were major fights and the 3rd Battalion, 11th Marines, moved in support of the 7th Marines. We moved into an area the infantry had just been through. The corpsmen and I followed a small stream—to reconnoiter—containing North Korean casualties—an incentive not to bathe in *that* stream. As we neared a very small village, a terrible smell assailed us. "Oh my God," I said, "There must be a lot of dead in there!"

One of the old hands said, "No, that's kimchee."

"What's kimchee?"

"The Korean national dish. They put cabbage, garlic, and hot peppers in a clay pot and bury the pot until the stuff ferments."

Late in the summer, the 11th Marines' regimental surgeon was transferred, and I was ordered to replace him. That job was dull and consisted mostly of keeping contact with the battalion surgeons and sending or signing reports prepared by the chief hospital corpsman. I wasn't there very long. The Division Surgeon had a policy of rotating doctors from line outfits to a rear echelon outfit about halfway through the one-year tour. By the end of summer all the doctors who joined at Inchon had rotated home. The Medical Battalion was left without an orthopedic surgeon. My orthopedic "training" consisted of three months of residency and about a year of "experience." But it was more than most, so I was sent to "A" Company, 1st Medical Battalion, in relief of Captain C. A. "Red" Stevenson, a trained orthopedic surgeon.

Each company was capable of loading, moving, and setting up in a new location in 12 hours. The three surgical companies were deployed in leapfrog fashion. The foremost was along the Main Supply Route just beyond enemy artillery range. The second was set up a mile or so rearward, and the third another mile or so back. Able Med was either set up along with the rearmost or still farther to the rear.

When the Division moved forward, the rearmost would evacuate its patients to a Med, saddle up, and move to the head of the queue and begin operating. That way definitive aid was never more than, say, three miles away from the fighting.

With the helicopter, aid was rapidly available for the critically wounded. During a time of heavy casualties, evacuation was to the forward company, and when it became swamped, to the next in line. When all three were full, casualties went to Able Med in the rear. If a regiment were going separately on a major assault, one of the medical companies would be detached to support it.

The more famous Army "MASH" units by my time had become so equipment-bound that it would take at least 48 hours to break down and set up. They had wood floors to their tents and an officers' club. They were far behind the lines, but with the helicopter to bring them patients, their doctors and nurses did surgery to be proud of. For instance, they showed us how to save legs by doing vein grafts to the femoral artery.

With the exodus of the well-trained surgeons from the Division, their slots were filled by young doctors, the most experienced of whom had three years of residency. It was a shame the Navy did not send trained men in to provide expert care for its wounded and teaching for the younger surgeons. Surgical teams were put together at Yokosuka, but they usually consisted of two gynecologists and a pediatrician and were of limited usefulness.

Even worse than the shortage of surgeons was the lack of anesthetists. That said, the green, partly trained surgeons performed commendably, and the survival and morbidity rate shows the kind of job they did. The survival rate of the wounded was better than in World War II. Skill was not all of it. We had whole blood and helicopter evacuation to thank as well.

Able Med had about 100 beds. Hospital tents were in 40-foot middle segments and end segments. By joining 40-foot segments you could have a ward stretching from Seoul to Pusan if you wanted to, but we had a manageable length of maybe three, plus ends. Each segment had an oil stove and a pipe stuck through the roof. We'd put up a surgical ward and parallel it a distance away with a medical ward. Forming a horseshoe between them was a long tent with the ER, triage, x-ray, and lab. Off this administrative wing were squad tents for major and minor surgery and orthopedics. The beds were folding canvas cots. At one time, policy was to keep any patient who could be returned to duty within 60 days. We added a convalescent tent parallel to the surgical ward.

Our chain of evacuation was by ambulance to the railhead at Taegu, from there by train to Pusan and the hospital ship, or to Yokosuka Naval Hospital. Another was by ambulance or helicopter to an airstrip, then to Yokosuka. At one point when we were near the east coast, a hospital ship lay offshore and we could evacuate to it by helicopter. Ships involved were *Consolation, Haven*, and *Repose.*

Because we were short of anesthetists, general anesthesia was reserved for belly and chest cases. Minor surgery and orthopedics were done under local. Sometimes I pumped in so much Xylocaine [Lidocaine] that I was sure the patient was going to have a reaction but none ever did.

Orthopedics and minor surgery overlapped and extremity wounds were so numerous that everybody had to do debridements, even the dentist if we were swamped. Patients would come into triage on a stretcher and usually stay on it during their whole tour through surgery. The stretcher would be placed between sawhorses in the triage area and in the O.R.. The triage doctor would go over them, get x-rays with our little portable machine, and assign them a priority or treatment order. He'd start fluids or blood and stabilize them for surgery.

My cases would come in, I'd examine them, look at the x-rays, scrub up in a "two-helmet" sink, and put on gloves. I wore a utility cap and mask and a rubber apron over my shirtless utilities. I usually did not wear a gown. Our kerosene autoclave couldn't keep up. I'd begin pumping Xylocaine and start debriding. The natural anesthesia of the recently wounded and age of the patients were in my favor. When finished, I'd put the bones in as good alignment as I could and apply a cast.

There are two inflexible rules, usually forgotten between wars. Debridement does not mean snipping away at wound edges with a scissors. The wound is laid wide open in all recesses, and entrance and exit wounds are connected. All dead and nonviable tissue is ruthlessly cut away. The wound is irrigated by the gallon and additional debridement done if necessary. The wound is covered with gauze and packed with fluffs of cotton waste and never closed. Accurate fracture reduction is not necessary, only a natural alignment. Somebody far away is going to have to deal with wound closure and definitive reduction. A cast is applied and immediately bivalved down to the skin.[3] You don't want the consequences of a swelling limb within an inflexible cast when a man is in transit.

Every patient in the chain of evacuation received intramuscular injections of penicillin and streptomycin at noon and midnight. The antibiotic was a supplement to the prevention of infection.

I neglected the rule about connecting entrance and exit wounds only once when I was green. A man was lying in his down sleeping bag when a shell fragment came through the tent, pierced the bag, and entered and exited his lateral thigh. I clipped away at the wounds of entrance and exit, squished a little saline at each end, and thought I'd save somebody some work. Several days later, foul smelling pus drained copiously from both wounds. I took him back to the O.R., opened the wound tract, and removed the down feathers that lined the tract. He did all right after that, and I learned a lesson I've never forgotten.

In August or September when the action stalled except for an occasional action to straighten the line, Able Med was directed to hold, and not evacuate, any patient who could be returned to duty within 60 days. This meant our census increased. We added a convalescent ward, and we had to secondarily close our wide-open debrided wounds.

Winter was coming and we knew how cold it was going to be. Regulations specified ample space between tents to lessen the danger of fire spreading. Someone had scrounged a machine called an aircraft engine pre-heater. A kerosene-fired flame produced heat and a gasoline-driven motor blew the heat along a reinforced canvas tube. We reasoned that with the heating tube running through the tents to supplement the oil stove in each tent section, we could keep the tents warm, especially if we moved the tents touching side by side. Fortunately, the assistant division commander came to inspect us, and Lt. Cmdr. Arv Henderson explained our plan. "The tents are marked 'Fire Retardant, General,'" as if that explained anything. Fortunately, he gave his permission and nobody was court-martialed.

One night when we were at chow, we heard a loud bang followed by a "poof." We thought we'd been hit. We ran out and saw that the heating machine had exploded, and because of its proximity to the back of a tent, set it on fire. Within five minutes the fire had run from one side of the tent horseshoe to the other. We could do nothing but stand and watch.

The ward corpsmen on duty were magnificent. They told the ambulatory patients to help the bed patients; most cut through the sidewalls of the tents. As the fire reached one of the oil stoves, it went up with a puff of flame and smoke. Oxygen tanks went off like large rockets. Patients were searched for ammunition before admission, but some had smuggled it in. It went up pyrotechnically.

All patients got out safely. The last one out was a Korean with one leg amputated and the other in a hip spica cast. He came out under his own power using his stump as a pusher. The only casualty was our CO, who burned his hands patting out a small flame on a tent rope.

Following the Able Med disaster, the entire patient population was transferred to a hospital ship offshore, to MASH units in the rear, and to Naval Hospital Yokosuka, Japan. Temporary tents were replaced so the unit could get back to partial operation. Within days, the Marine Engineer Battalion arrived and reconstructed Able Med with semipermanent buildings. No more tents.

* * *

Acting Battalion Surgeon

Donald Kent began his career during World War II as an Army enlisted man. He was then sent to an Army Special Training Program (ASTP) unit at Yale for a semester, and accepted into medical school. But until there was room for him, he worked as an x-ray technician at the Fitzsimons Army General Hospital in Denver, Colorado. By the time he finished an accelerated course at the University of Nebraska Medical School, the war was over and he was discharged from the Army.

After just a year in private practice, Dr. Kent applied for a Reserve commission in the Navy. In 1951, he went to the Naval Medical School in Bethesda, Maryland, where he studied tropical diseases and public health. Then he took an intensified course in aerospace medicine in Pensacola, Florida, and a five-week submarine medicine course in New London, Connecticut. After more training at the Field Medical Service School, Camp Lejeune, North Carolina, it looked as though he was now prepared for an operational assignment in any branch of Navy medicine. At the time, he recalls, they were really having a hard time getting people to volunteer for Korea. Without much further thought, he made his choice—the 1st Marine Division.

I was immediately sent to Camp Pendleton and got there in time to get with a replacement draft that was on its way to Korea. We learned to fire weapons, went on field exercises, and made landings with the amphibious force. We learned how to set up aid stations and perform emergency medicine in the field. It was a pretty good orientation. And with all my medical training, I was well oriented—more than most people who went over.

We were on a troop transport under operational blackout all the way so it was pretty much a quiet trip. We stopped in Kobe, Japan, where we got rid of all our personal effects. All the gear we had with us was replenished with whatever else we needed in the field, and we spent three or four days there. I was a senior medical officer with the replacement draft so I had to go through all the people in the draft to see that all of their shots were up to date. If they weren't, we took care of them right there in Kobe.

After about three or four days there we headed out to Korea and landed in Pusan. Our whole replacement draft was put in a tent camp. About two days later we were all flown up north just south of the 38th Parallel.

At first, I was assigned to the engineer shore party but was only there for a couple of days because they still hadn't decided where I would remain. Then an opening came up for battalion surgeon for the 3rd Battalion, 7th Marines, an infantry battalion. The 7th Marines were then in reserve so I joined them and got acquainted with the officers of the staff and with my corpsmen.

The Punchbowl operation [August–September 1951] was to kick off in about five days. We were to be the lead battalion and lead regiment for the operation. We went into action and, after about a week, I decided I should be as far forward as I could get with my aid station. I took a corpsman and a chaplain, and we deployed ourselves maybe half a mile behind the line of engagement and about a hundred yards from the MLR. The aid station was just a dugout in the side of a hill. We didn't have a table to operate on. We worked on a stretcher on the ground.

We were under fire almost every day, and constantly seeing people who were hit. I did some emergency surgeries on the frontline, including a tracheotomy on one fellow. He was hit with a shrapnel wound to his neck. All the tissue around his trachea was swollen and his airway was obstructed. I made the incision and inserted an emergency tracheotomy tube without anesthesia. We actually saved the guy's life.

I had a small surgical kit, plasma, bandages, and morphine. And that was it. The main thing was to triage people. There were only two ways of getting the wounded off the line. One was helicopter and the other was to put them on a stretcher and carry them back by Korean stretcher-bearers.

We had a Marine radioman with us at the frontline. If we needed a helicopter, he would call in our location and they would send us one. Every time we moved, we would set up an area in a defile area where it would be safe for a helicopter to land. We would have provided first aid as much as we could, administering morphine to control pain and stop any bleeding, and would have started plasma. The helicopter would then pick up the patient and fly him back to Able Med.

Able Med was probably four miles back behind the line. A man could be hit, given first aid within minutes, be on a helicopter in half an hour, and on an operating table within an hour. It was a fast evacuation and fast care.

The helicopters were the little Bell helicopters with a pod on each side that you could put the stretcher in, and there was a cover that went over it. You could evacuate two at a time and, almost always, we had more than one.

Most of the injuries we treated were shrapnel from either mortars or artillery. During the Punchbowl there were a lot of casualties. We evacuated maybe 30 or 40 a day.

Even though I had only had a rotating internship and wasn't really a surgeon, I was acting surgeon. In fact, I was the battalion surgeon. That was my title. I wished I had more surgical training, but it wasn't available at that stage. There were instances when I did what a corpsman probably would not have been able to do. But the average things we did such as stopping bleeding—clamping off bleeding vessels—he could have done.

In November of '51, I was transferred back to the regiment—the 7th Marines. This was a couple of miles behind the frontline. We had a tent that was sort of semipermanent because the regiment was in a semipermanent position. I had a chief hospital corpsman and six other corpsmen. The chain of evacuation was like this: Somebody would be injured on the frontline or somebody would be sick at battalion level. They would be transferred back to the regiment, and the regiment would decide where they would be evacuated. One choice was what they called "collecting and clearing companies." A collecting and clearing company was a small mobile hospital that could do some emergency surgery. It could do more advanced care than could be done on the frontline, but not the more extensive type of surgery that was possible at what was called "Able Med." Able Med was basically the division hospital.

They had all the surgical specialties at Able Med, including a general surgeon, a thoracic surgeon, an eye surgeon, and, at times, even a neurosurgeon was assigned. Able Med was in a fixed position.

I was at Easy Med for about a week. We were behind a hill. On the other side of the hill toward the frontline was the Marine artillery battalion. One day our artillery battalion had been firing toward the North Korean and Chinese lines. In the morning I heard what we called an "air burst." That's when a shell goes off in the air. An air burst could mean one of two things. Either our outgoing fire had gone off prematurely or else the enemy was firing at us—what we call "fire for effect." All of a sudden another round went off a little bit closer, and I said, "Enemy fire! Evacuate the tent!"

I had about half a dozen patients in the tent at the time. I picked up and carried one of the more serious ones who couldn't go by himself, and got him to our bunker. Then I went back into the tent. By this time the corpsmen were starting to evacuate the walking wounded. Some of them had gotten a few patients out into the bunker. I went back into the tent and picked up another one of the wounded. I had just gotten out of the tent, maybe ten yards away, when an artillery round landed right on the tent and absolutely disintegrated the whole thing. There were still two patients and one corpsman in there and they were all killed. I was far enough away but got shrapnel in my left arm. The firing continued so there was nothing we could do at that time except lie there until the thing was over.

I couldn't make it to the bunker because I was afraid to leave where I was. When things calmed down a little, I went back up and looked in the tent. There was nothing I could do there.

When things were quiet they got me into an ambulance with another patient. The two of us were evacuated to Easy Med where they debrided and dressed my wounds but told me I needed further treatment. I had three through-and-through wounds of my upper humerus—my upper shoulder. Also, one of the pieces of shrapnel had taken off a little piece of periosteum of the humerus. It wasn't really a fracture.

I was then evacuated to Able Med where they finished the debridement and decided that I didn't need a cast so they put me in a sling. They told me they would treat me there and then keep me as staff for the rest of my assignment. So I ended up in Able Med where I worked as a staff physician. I started out as a general medical officer, and then ran the eye clinic. I became a makeshift ophthalmologist for a while. Before I left Able Med, I also acted as the head of the Internal Medicine Division and finally became executive officer of the hospital company.

We could do most anything at Able Med, including open chest work and any kind of orthopedics. However, we didn't do any definitive surgery there. This was still a facility where we provided basic surgery before sending our patients to a hospital ship or Yokosuka for definitive care. We only held people we felt were going back to the line.

* * *

"This Was Not M*A*S*H"

Hermes Grillo attended Harvard Medical School under Navy auspices during the last days of World War II. When he completed medical school at twenty-three, he began surgical residency at Massachusetts General Hospital in Boston. Three years later when the Korean War broke out, Dr. Grillo had become a civilian again. He now had four choices: the Public Health Service, the Air Force, the Army, or Navy. "For someone interested in surgery the Army made sense, but I liked the Navy and I figured I'd do two years... I'd spend one year at sea, and I like the sea. I pictured myself on a ship in the Mediterranean, of course—naturally the sun, the Med squadron, and then a year in a Naval hospital doing something moderately interesting."

After a very short tour at Naval Hospital Chelsea, Massachusetts, where he worked in neurosurgery, Grillo received orders to the Fleet Marine Force. That could mean only one outcome. His dream of serving aboard ship in the Med was over.

Following orientation at Camp Lejeune's Field Medical School, Lt.(j.g.) Grillo went with the 1st Marine Division to Korea. His introduction to the war was immediate and dramatic.

They got us together on the airfield and told us we'd be flying up to the forward area. They said the weather was bad and weren't sure they could land but would try. The weather opened just enough to drop in through clouds onto a gravel strip. We got into an open truck and it was pouring by that point. This would have been the end of February or early April [1951]. It took about four hours to finally get to the forward area, and by that time it was night.

I reported to the commander, who turned out to be Cmdr. [Richard] Lawrence, head of the medical battalion 1st MARDIV. He was in a dugout with sandbags, a kerosene lantern, and a four-day growth of beard. Artillery shells were whistling around, and we could hear the crackle of machine-gun fire. It was really active. The sky was lighting up and I remember thinking, "Geez, it's like a World War I movie." It was kind of exciting.

They wanted doctors. In a sense, I think, nobody looked at what we did or had as backgrounds. So we were just sent up, undifferentiated, as a mass of medical officers.

The commander asked about my background. I said, "Three and a half years of surgical residency, sir."

He looked at me, his eyes got big, and he said, "All surgery?"

I told him yes.

And he said, "Company D."

I didn't know what that meant and so I picked up my pack and my rifle.

You couldn't get there walking so they jeeped me up to an old rice paddy. It was dark and raining and pouring. I got to a tent and that was Co. D. It was a squad tent with a kerosene lantern hanging there. I spoke to the first person I saw sitting on his cot. He told me the commanding officer was over there and he jerked his finger to the rear. I walked to a cot at the back, and I could just see a gray rotund belly lying there. I couldn't see a face. I had no idea what I was going to be doing. I thought that I might be helping some red-hot board surgeon. That seemed pretty good.

"I was told to report here, sir." There was silence. So I just stood there for a while. And then a voice with no face attached to it came out of the dark dripping with sarcasm.

"So you're the new surgeon." I quickly figured that I'm the surgeon here, not just an assistant. I was it, I thought. Well, that didn't sound too bad so I just stood there thinking that I don't know what kind of surgical work they do here; maybe it's first aid. I said nothing more; I didn't know what to say.

Finally the voice said, "How much training have *you* had?"

I said, "Three and a half years, sir."

There was dead silence, and then the voice said, "Jesus Christ, another one!"

And then I got a stream of vituperation. Not foul language but: "These kids out here are getting wounded bad, they're getting all shot up, their guts are getting shot up. We don't need boys out here; we need men. We need board-trained surgeons. We need experienced surgeons. We don't need a bunch of kids like you."

I thought to myself, "It's cold up here. It's wet. It's dangerous. There's machine-gun fire out there. It's muddy. This guy sounds like a sonofabitch." I felt like saying, "If you don't want me, I'll go home." I knew better than to say that so I just stood there.

After a while he cooled down and that was the end of that. Somebody showed me where my cot was and I stowed my stuff. About three minutes later a corpsman stuck his head in the tent flap and said, "Guy with a belly wound out here."

I walked across to the "hospital" tent and found a kid with a belly wound. I think it was a bunch of fragment wounds. He wasn't in bad shape. He wasn't in shock; he just needed to be fixed. I looked at him quickly. You don't do much of a physical. They are eighteen years old, healthy, hard as nails, and they've had a recent wound. That was the whole history for every one of them.

So I went back in. I didn't know the drill. I had no idea what was going on. I didn't even know who anybody was. I went back to the commanding officer and said, "The patient has an abdominal wound, sir, and he needs to be taken care of," or words to that effect. Again there was dead silence. So I wondered, maybe this is like a residency and he's the boss. So I said, "Do you want to check him over, sir?" I just felt we had to get off dead center.

The voice said, "Check him over? Hell no! You want anesthesia, I'll give you anesthesia. You don't want it, I'll stay in the sack."

I remember a tremendous feeling of relief. First of all, I now had information. I knew he was the anesthetist. And the second thing was I now felt this guy, who I thought at this point was a sonofabitch, which he wasn't, was going to be off my back with regard to medical decisions. I felt OK. I don't mind making my own decisions; he won't be around second-guessing me because obviously we are not going to get along. I said, "I want anesthesia." So he clomped out and went in and put the kid to sleep very effectively, very efficiently. I just went to work. There was nothing to it after three and half years of surgical training. I just zipped the kid open and cleaned him up as best I could. The lights were terrible and the equipment was terrible, but we managed. I sewed up the holes, debrided them, and made sure there were no other things that I overlooked, and then sewed him up. It didn't take very long and it went very well. He watched very closely, didn't say word.

When I finished, he said, "I think we're going to get along."

I consider him a friend—he's dead now, poor guy. His name was Dan Pino.

After a few days, he began to warm up, even though he was not a man of many words. He was very laconic, I would say, but a very good guy—very well motivated. I said, "Cmdr. Pino, if I run into some problems I can't handle or don't quite know what to do with, is there somebody I can call? Who can I call?" We had a field telephone.

He looked at me thoughtfully for a moment, then shook his head and said very sadly, "There's nobody."

I couldn't understand that. This was a division, a reinforced division. I don't know whether it was twenty-five thousand men with tanks and artillery and all the rest. And I thought, "I'm *the* surgeon for this division? This has gotta be crazy." Well, it turned out that I had the most experience of anyone in that division.

The first place we were was someplace south of Inje, a small city up toward the [38th] Parallel. We were actually on the side of a gently sliding little hill, which went down into a rice paddy. At that point it was very small. When wounded men came in and if they were in good shape, they would put the stretchers on the ground with the head up the hill. If they were in shock, they would put them with their heads down the hill. We had one operating tent, another debriding tent, a minor operating room, and then a couple of squad tents for the post-ops who were evacuated very promptly to Company A—the medical company. If they were minor wounds, they would go back down there until they got well enough to go back to the front. If they had major wounds, we kept them until they were stable. And then we tried to move them out as fast as possible because our conditions were terrible.

That summer [1951] they started the so-called Panmunjom truce talks. We actually had our heaviest casualties that fall when we decided to "straighten the line." We had a few thousand casualties in a couple of days. It was a slaughterhouse because the Marines went up the hill against bunkers where the North Koreans were dug in. Occasionally things would quiet down a little bit, and then we would have another great run. With our limited personnel, it didn't take long to absolutely saturate us.

The medical organization was like this: Theoretically, you had battalion surgeons, battalion aid stations. Then you had collecting and clearing companies—C, D, and E. Then there was the base medical company, Company A, and that was supposed to be on the beach. And from the beach, patients would evacuate to a hospital ship where they would have surgery. That was the theory.

We were close to the 38th Parallel at that point. We eventually ended up near the Punchbowl north of the parallel. The hospital then was in Pusan, a long way down. Obviously, if you tried to move the wounded down there, many would never get there. As you know, the helicopters were helpful. But for the largest percentage of wounded, the helicopters were theoretical. First of all, you had the mountains. Even on good days, the fog often didn't clear until ten in the morning.

Most of the time ambulances brought down the wounded. In the mountains, roads used to be bulldozed out of the side of a mountain or hill. Sometimes the road would wash out in heavy rains, or sometimes troops or tanks would be moving and the ambulances had to wait because they were not first priority.

So, medical evacuation had been reorganized. A couple of the collecting/clearing companies were made into hospital units. When I was there, there were two. Ours was Dog Company and then there was Easy Med Company. Those two were made into surgical units of a sort. The advantage was that we were very close because theoretically we supported one regiment. There were two regiments up and one back in reserve. Ours was the 5th Marines. We also had a second regiment of Korean Marines, and we gave medical support to them because they had no other medical support. They were hellions, a bunch of youngsters who were determined to do anything that the U.S. Marines could do and do it better. They got into all kinds of trouble.

We also treated anything that came down the line—U.S. Army troops because often we would have an Army group next to the Marines, the next unit over. Their collecting and clearing was sometimes to the rear of where we were doing surgery. If they had a really badly wounded man, they would not send him farther back to the rear to a MASH, which was many miles back. A MASH supported a division rather than a regiment. They would send the patient up to the front to us to be operated on because we were fifteen minutes away and the other MASH might be several hours back.

The hospital ships weren't of any immediate use. What they did do, as far as I understand it, was this. After we debrided the relatively minor wounds, we would get them out the next day, or even the same day, in ambulances back to Company A, where they held them. The worst ones they eventually shipped down to the hospital ship. We would keep the severely wounded men until they were stable, which was usually five to seven days. And then we'd get them the hell out of there, and they

would go back to the hospital ship. Some of them made it directly to Yokosuka
Naval Hospital after they had been triaged. Most of the severely wounded ones
eventually ended up in Yokosuka. One of my friends from Mass General, a year
behind me in residency, was on the surgical staff there. He saw a lot of my patients
after they got there. He could later tell me about cases and what happened to them.
That was the general triage. But the definitive surgery was done in our units. There
were five doctors but I was the only surgeon.

Basically we had only one major operating room—and that was mine. I processed
the wounded as fast as I could. They did work out a system later on, where they
could direct helicopters either to Easy Med or to us, depending upon who was
or was not bombed with cases at the time. Occasionally a company would get
overwhelmed. I think it was Company A, at one point, that suddenly got hit during
an attack. They were overwhelmed and they called us on the field telephone. Pino
said OK we'd come down. So he and I got in a jeep and drove down there. They
set us up in a tent, and we just operated for what seemed to me several days steady.
I never did know. Sometimes I would step out and it was day and other times it
was night. You'd go out and pee, and then they'd bring you a hamburger or a
sandwich and some coffee and I'd go back. I was only twenty-six or twenty-seven
at that time. I actually got to a point where I thought I would drop from exhaustion,
but we just couldn't stop. In my own unit, I couldn't ever stop since there was no
alternate.

In the winter the tents were cold as hell. Each had a little kerosene stove, and
you had to have a man watching it all the time so the tent wouldn't catch fire. I
went to the new commanding officer, Cmdr. George Tarr, and said, "George, we've
got to do something about these tents. We need to get some canvas and double-wall
them and make them a little warmer. Finally he got so irritated with me he said,
"Do anything you want to do."

I went to our supply man and got a bunch of little medicine bottles filled with
ethyl alcohol. We only used ethyl. The Navy was realistic and knew personnel
would drink the stuff no matter what it was. If you gave them isopropyl, they'd get
sick and poison themselves so we used ethyl. That way they couldn't get anything
but drunk. Anyway, I had them fill up a bunch of these four-ounce bottles with
alcohol, put them in a bag, got a truck, and started down the Main Supply Route.

We got to an Army unit and I found the supply sergeant, and I told him about
all these poor, wounded Marines freezing up there near the front. He said, "Geez,
Doc, I wish I could help you but you know there's nothing I can do."

I pulled out a bottle of alcohol, slammed it down on the counter, and said, "Well,
sergeant, thank you for your understanding anyway and maybe you can use this."

He said, "What's that?"

I said, "Ethyl alcohol."

"Can you drink it?"

"Goddamn right you can drink it. You mix it up with grapefruit juice and you've got yourself one helluva drink."

His eyes brightened and he said, "Just a minute, Doc, I just remembered." He went in the back room and came out with a pile of blankets four feet high and then said, "Got any more of that stuff?"

This scenario, straight out of "Mr. Roberts," was repeated at about three different units down that line. We'd stop in and get the same story, "Can't help you." We got back and the guys went to work and they double-walled the tents. By that evening they were sitting around in their skivvy shirts.

It was that kind of constant business where you did the best you could. People pitched in and worked hard. The only thing I wished we had was more trained personnel and some more equipment so we could do a proper job.

I got the flu some time that winter and I was running a temperature of about 102 or 103. I would lie in my cot and they would get a Marine on the table and then would call me. I'd go through the snow and operate on the guy and then go back and lie down again until the next one came along. There wasn't anyone else you could call on. Unfortunately, nobody ever came through who had surgical training. It was that kind of situation. One advantage was that we were so close to the front that I'm sure we probably saved people who would never have made it back to the rear.

That was the principal concept that various consultants came up with from their experience in World War II. Do definitive surgery—not patches and dressings and such—as close to the front as possible so that you can immediately treat casualties who are bleeding massively, who have guts blown out and so on. That was the MASH concept. But, of course, the MASHs, since they supported at least a division, had to be farther back since lines of evacuation are perpendicular to the front. We, on the other hand, could be right up close because, theoretically, we were only dealing with a regiment. That was an advantage and it worked out pretty well, I think.

Equipment-wise, it was so bad that it taught me a tremendous amount about improvisation, which has served me well for the rest of my career. We had a miserable little kerosene sterilizer. We had an operating table. It was a small collapsible metal thing that was so low to the ground we stood it on ammunition cases to get it up to a height where I could use it and not have to break my back. You could not adjust it in any way. You just had to put the patient on it and then move him around.

We had plenty of sterile supplies, linens and such. We had no true operating room lights. We had a bulb hanging from a cord over the table. I stole a reflector from an engineering searchlight and put that over the top of the bulb, which made it a little better. I borrowed an engineer's searchlight once and it was so hot it cooked and desiccated the tissues so I got rid of that in a hurry. Initially, I learned to operate with a flashlight clipped to the back of my belt. Sometimes at night the lights would go out; the generators were not dependable, and everyone would be stumbling around and I would say, "Reach in my back pocket and you will find a flashlight." And somebody would fumble around. I remember finishing a bowel anastomosis with this flashlight.

We had a very thin supply of instruments in terms of variations and variety. But you know you can do most of that kind of surgery with ordinary instruments. We had no suction machines. So when I had a belly full of feces and exudate and twigs and blood, I would just scoop it out with my hand onto the dirt floor. And then we would take big abdominal pads and just wipe the belly out, pour saline in, and clean it out as best we could. If there was a mess of bleeding welling up, all you could do was to put pressure on things and then slowly work your way in because there was no suction of any sort available. For deep wounds, you were way down somewhere in the depths.

There were no deep abdominal retractors. There were all these miserable little things a few centimeters long. I took some 155mm brass shell cases—which are big and heavy and long—and I drew on them outlines of retractors that I wanted. On a piece of paper I drew the curve I wanted and we took them down to the engineers. They cut these for me from the heavy brass, bent and filed them, and these are what we used. They weighed a ton. I wish I had taken one back for a souvenir, but I had to leave them there for other guys to use. But because we had no big abdominal retractors, we had to use these things and they were very helpful.

One night a Marine stepped on a mine and blew a hole in his perineum. His urethra was a mess, and I thought I would try to put a catheter in before I reconstructed his urethra. Fortunately, in my residency, I'd had a little bit of everything—neurosurgery, urology, orthopedics—so I tackled all these things. I just looked around for a stilette but couldn't find one. So I just took a piece of bailing wire off an ammunition case that we had in the corner, and I bent that around in the right shape, wiped it off with alcohol, and put it through the catheter and that became a stilette.

To my knowledge, I think I did the first vascular graft ever done in the U.S. Armed Forces. I believe it was April of 1951.[4] This kid came in with a femoral artery shot out. I couldn't bear just tying off the artery. I remembered a procedure I'd seen at Mass General one day. Robert Linton, who was our vascular surgeon, did an excision of a popliteal aneurysm and the patient's foot turned white and cold. He turned the patient over, took a piece of saphenous vein, and put a graft in. I remembered thinking, "Why didn't they do this in World War II?" All they did then was ligate arteries or try Blakemore tubes, which didn't work.

I decided that the only thing I could do was to take a piece of saphenous vein and put a graft in. I used eye instruments, some fine silk suture material, and some heparin. It stayed patent but the patient eventually died from renal shutdown. I didn't feel very good because the patient had died, but surgically that graft was important.

They shipped us blood, which was all universal donor or blood with substances to neutralize the antibodies. There was no cross-matching. The blood was just poured in. And we used huge amounts of it, sometimes six or eight [units] for a guy who was exsanguinating when he arrived. The problem was that there was a custom. As new blood came in, each unit to the rear would take the new blood, put it in their refrigerator, and send the old stuff forward. So the stuff we got—where a lot of blood was really used—was full of stringy clots and it looked awful. I don't know how many people we killed with that blood, probably not too many; they seemed to survive it. We had a refrigerator and kept it cool with a generator. We had all the blood we needed. There was never a shortage.

This was not *M*A*S*H*. *M*A*S*H* was very well equipped in comparison. *M*A*S*H* was not bad. *M*A*S*H* had good equipment, good lighting, x-ray machines, and a corps of trained surgeons who were at my level. And these were the second-order people. They had board-trained Army surgeons. They had nurses. They had endless supplies and they had staffs that didn't have to work around the clock because they had enough people; they could be on rotations. Of course, when they got bombed, everyone would all pitch in, but normally you'd be on duty, you'd be off duty. We had no on-duty/off-duty for the doctors.

We were on duty and when it got very busy, we just went and went and went. There was never even a question in my mind of ever stopping. I didn't feel I had the option. There's a guy on the table and you have to do something for him. We had enough corpsmen so they worked in shifts. But I remember one time when we were absolutely overwhelmed, just working away. I looked up and saw this corpsman—a good guy—who worked in the operating room. I said, "You know you've been on for twenty-four hours now."

He looked at me and said, "Well, we figured if the doctors can do it, we can do it."

These were the good things you saw; these fellows felt that they were obligated, too. And the morale went zooming up after we got things moving and better organized.

We moved about four or five times while [I was in Korea], and I can't even tell you where. It was always some valley. The commanding officer would go up in a jeep with the Medical Service Corps officer, and they'd find a place in the area close enough to the front. It would be a reasonably safe place, sometimes behind a hill or in a little flat place but near the MSR so they could get to us quickly. We first started in a rice paddy and then we moved to Inje, then up to a valley that was just over a ridge from the 5th Marines. They brought the wounded back over the hill.

Then we moved again another time. The final place got pretty well set up once the talks started in Panmunjom. Later we got wooden decks for the operating tents, which we hadn't had. By this time we had figured out a way to bring jeeps up so we could hook up to their generators if we lost power at night. We even had screens for the hot weather late that fall. Before that I always had one extra corpsman stand at the table keeping the flies off. It was aesthetically troublesome to me to be sewing up someone's intestine and have a fly sit on it. This didn't seem to do anyone any harm—the patients did all right—but it was very upsetting to me.

When I think about it, the only obligation the Navy Medical Department had in the Korean War was the Marine division. Oh, the Navy ships went up and down the coast and fired a few shells and occasionally an artillery observer went ashore. They had twenty-five thousand men there getting shot at, and out of the whole huge complex of the Navy Medical Department, they couldn't muster up two board surgeons—that would have been the minimum need—or even a couple of more guys like myself, and there were lots of them. When I got back to St. Albans Naval Hospital, the place was just loaded with surgeons of all types—regular Navy, Reservists, and so on. You would also think they could get somebody who had at least one year of anesthesia residency.

I left Korea just before Christmas near the close of '51. When I got the information that I could leave the next day—my number had come up—I had this tremendous sense of relief. But I was so involved in this thing and thought we were doing a good job. You have this feeling. You've got a job to do here and you're doing it well—and who's going to take over? Then I thought, "You've gotta be crazy. Leave when you can."

Notes
[1]James Forrestal, Secretary of Defense.
[2]Dr. Arioli was the only Navy physician killed in action during the Korean War.
[3]Bivalving means cutting the cast hemispherically into two halves to allow for expansion.
[4]According to Dr. Otto Apel, he and Dr. John Coleman, chief surgeon of the 8076 MASH, began performing vein grafts on patients in the summer of 1951.

11

Prisoner of War

The Chinese showed up in the middle of the night, preceded by a thundering artillery barrage. Marines defending an outpost a thousand yards beyond the MLR (Main Line of Resistance) hunkered down in their underground shelters. Ignoring a minefield and barbed wire entanglements, the enemy approached the American positions at a dead run firing burp guns and hurling satchel charges and concussion grenades. During forty-five minutes of hand-to-hand combat, thirty-two enlisted men and one officer held out against a force that outnumbered them nearly four to one, but eventually they were forced to withdraw to the safety of the MLR. Not all made it before the communists regained control of the barren, pock-marked hilltop that had already changed hands several times. There were dead and wounded—and there were prisoners.

Every warrior's worst nightmare was falling into enemy hands. The first moments of captivity were the most terrifying. Disarmed and helpless, the captured were at the mercy of their captors. As they struggled to comprehend what was now expected of them as prisoners, the ruthless Chinese soldiers prodded them to the rear at gunpoint. Their future was not promising. This was a cruel enemy, notorious for starving prisoners, withholding medical treatment, and practicing a sadistic form of psychological torture. As the reality of the situation began to sink in, each man dealt with his own level of despair.

During the Korean War, 225 Marines and 35 Navy personnel became prisoners of war. Three were Navy medical personnel: HN (Hospitalman) Thomas H. Waddill, HN Thomas A. Scheddel, and HM3 (Hospital Corpsman third class) Billy Penn.

* * *

HN Thomas Waddill of Charlie Company, 3rd Battalion, 5th Marines, saw his first firefight on 25 March 1953 and, in a letter, pulled no punches telling his parents what combat was like. He was captured the following day.

Dear Folks,

Well here it is 2:00 in the morning and I am on the phone in the platoon CP [command post]. It is raining awful hard outside and that is what everyone hates. The trenches cave in and get about three feet deep in old red mud. I just came off a three-night ambush affair. We set up in a rice paddy just across from Goony land at sundown and didn't secure until 12:00 each night. It wasn't too cold. I was so scared I was warm. We were set in in the Goony trench line and we found potato masher hand grenades all over the place. Baker Company pulled off a daylight raid on them. Got just across the rice paddy to our left. They had seven killed and 54 wounded. A corpsman that came out in my draft got hit in the legs by shrapnel, but he is going to be okay.

Dad, I am going to tell you what my job consists of. Any time a patrol ambush or anything like that goes out in front of the barb [sic] wire, a corpsman goes with them. I go along just like any other Marine except I carry a stretcher and my first aid kit. Since I have to protect myself if we get into a fire fight I carry a .45 pistol and usually three or four fragmentation hand grenades. I feel just like an owl since I do my work at night. Sometimes it is so dark that you would have to practically run right over a Goony before either of you could see each other. Since the Gooks have started wearing black uniforms it really makes it rough.

I got my baptism of fire the other night. We were going out to set up an ambush and had to go down this deep draw. Well old Luke was waiting for us with four burp guns and three machine guns. It was real dark. I was about eighth man back. Luke cut loose when our lead man was about five feet from him. They killed him instantly, wounded three more before we clobbered him with Thompson machine guns and grenades. You could hear the Gooks running around and hear them jabbering like mad. They holler like that because they know that it shakes you up and it does. We got everyone patched and got them back to the Forward Aid station behind our lines. For a while I was really scared but when I started taking care of the guys who got hit, I didn't even think about old Luke. That's the only fire fight I have been in, and I hope it is the last because they are really bad business.

I got your package with the salmon, olives and pickles and everything else. You really did pick just what I want and everything was delicious. I haven't got the Mexican chow yet but I am hungrily awaiting it. That's about it for now so good morning from Korea.

Love,
Tom

The next day, 26 March, the situation turned sour for the 3rd Battalion, 5th Marines. A sustained, heavy artillery bombardment generated many casualties and, for the first time in Korea, three Navy hospital corpsmen fell into communist hands. Besides Tom Waddill, who was captured at outpost Reno, HM3 Billy R. Penn, who was helping defend Vegas, also became a POW. The horrors of close combat and subsequent captivity scarred Penn and his comrades for the rest of their lives.

Following his repatriation in the first exchange of sick and wounded prisoners known as "Little Switch" in April 1953, Penn received medical treatment and then went back to the States.[1] "Three weeks after returning home, I was back at work in a Navy hospital in Pensacola. I had three surgeries on my right eye and a lot of 'sandpapering' to remove some of the superficial shrapnel. Even today, sometimes while shaving, I'll tear up a razor blade when it hits the shrapnel."

In March 1995, at the request of his friend and former Commandant of the Marine Corps, Gen. Robert H. Barrow, Penn chronicled his experiences as a prisoner of war. What tortures he endured at the hands of his captors and the atrocities he witnessed are very disturbing and almost too horrible to contemplate. For forty-five years the memories tormented him, affecting sleep, marriage, family, and profession. Writing down those recollections was an effort to help salve the wounds that never healed.

My tour of duty as a hospital corpsman attached to the Fleet Marine Force started off on a rather ominous date. The fifty of us from Pendleton Marine Base arrived in Korea on Friday the 13th in February of 1953. Even though my tenure in Korea, North and South, was short compared to some of the experiences of the Vietnam POWs, it seemed like a lifetime on occasion. I think maybe the Vietnam POWs were a little more prepared than we were then. As you know, the Chinese and the North Koreans had never heard of the Geneva Convention.

After landing in Seoul, they were transferring us at night to a rest area, which was approximately three miles behind our MLR. They gave each one of us an empty M1 to carry up there; however, I found one clip of ammunition and took it with me.

On the way up with about three of us in a truck, enemy mortar fire was really getting close. The truck driver told us to get out and get away from the truck. I started running and I guess I ran a hundred yards or so. After the mortar shells stopped, they started calling my name, and when the driver realized where I was, he told me not to move. It seems that I had run out in the middle of a minefield, and they had to get the engineers to come and get me. I was really starting off in good fashion.

Our main jobs for the first two to three weeks were patrols between the rest areas and our MLRs. There were a lot of artillery shells day and night. Finally we moved up to our MLR to replace a company on the MLR when that company pulled a daylight raid on a hilltop called Oongot. They suffered a 90 percent casualty rate. The first casualty I took care of was Geronimo, an American Indian. It seemed like all American Indians were nicknamed either Cochise or Geronimo.

Our company had to go out that night after the daylight raid to pick up the dropped equipment the Marines had left. We went out again the next night, farther up the hill, and I found the Korean dolls I now have in a Chinese machine gun bunker. We stayed on the MLR because the other company had such a high casualty rate. We made two patrols at night, and I was the only corpsman so therefore I had the honor of going on both patrols. On one patrol we were ambushed on the way back. I had one bad casualty I was trying to drag back when I ran into some Chinese, and the casualty and I lay in a ditch that night for a long time.

After the Chinese left, I heard Roscoe Woodard calling for me. He had come back for us. Thank God for Woody! Woody and I had long talks about home. He was from Lucedale, Mississippi. I was from McComb, Mississippi. We talked about home, families, and the Corps. I seems that Woody already had a couple of Purple Hearts. He had been wounded twice before, was in the hospital for three months, and elected to stay in Korea rather than to go stateside.

Finally I was attached to the 5th Marines, 3rd Battalion, H Company. One afternoon we got word that a corpsman was needed on Vegas. I volunteered to go. We had three outposts between our MLR and the Chinese MLR—Reno, Vegas, and Carson. They were so named because they felt it was such a gamble to be out there. I knew that Woody was already out there as a machine gunner.

On the way out, a lot of incoming mortar and big stuff were hitting close. How could they see us? We were on the backside of a tall hill. Incoming was getting heavier when we got to the trenches on Vegas. I went straight to the command bunker when the artillery really intensified. I was in the bunker when I could hear somebody calling for a corpsman. I was taking care of a Marine when two Chinese jumped on me in the trench. They were like ants, all over us. One stuck a bayonet through my left leg above the ankle and I couldn't move; he couldn't get the bayonet out, and I saw his finger on the trigger and his gun clicked. They had taught us that if you ever had a bayonet in somebody and you couldn't get it out, to fire the rifle, and the recoil would help pull it out.

I knew I was about to lose a foot. He started to cock his rifle with the bolt action when I got my .45 and shot him in the head. It moved him about three feet down the trench. I was an expert with a .45. At boot camp they kept trying to get me to stay on with the Marine Pistol Team. Thoughts of that have gone through my mind since that time. The Chinese are so small; they look just like ants with a ten-inch waist. They were all over us. They had run up on the hill with their own artillery still firing.

I was able to remove the bayonet and rifle still in my leg and started pulling the Marine into the command bunker. I was hit in the left knee superficially with shrapnel, took a shot by burp gun in the right shoulder, a through and through wound. I didn't really know about the shoulder until later when I saw how much blood I had lost.

A bayonet in the right lower back glanced off my flak jacket. It barely scratched my skin, but it scared the devil out of me. As I turned, my elbow caught him in the throat, he fell, and I jumped on him. The adrenaline was flowing so I'm not really sure about him, but I hit him so many times he did not move after I got up. This is very difficult to write.

They were all over us. I picked up an entrenchment tool and started swinging. I hit one in the neck, and the way his body was shaking on the ground I thought I had decapitated him. I had a flashback of wringing a chicken's neck at home.

Dead Chinese all over. Our machine gunners and Marines had really done a job on the first wave of Chinese. I had been told that the first wave of Chinese had the weapons and that most of the second wave did not have weapons. They were supposed to get their weapons from the fallen first wave. Everyone was in hand-to-hand combat. A Chinese and I were "involved." He had me on the ground with a bayonet over his head driving it toward me. I reached up and gouged out both his eyes as we rolled over. I remember seeing him running around screaming. I saw Woody standing outside his machine gun bunker swinging his M2 [automatic carbine] like a baseball bat. Trying to get another Marine back to the command bunker, I was jumped again by a Chinese and I beat him unconscious with a rock. I started out of the command bunker again—the door was only about four feet tall—and as I stooped to get out, I was hit by a rifle butt on my helmet. Reflexively, I raised my .45 and when it went off, it was on the tip of his nose. I'll never forget the expression on his face as the .45 went off, or the feeling I had seeing what power it had at pointblank range.

I backed into the command bunker seeing what looked like a thousand Chinese over Vegas, even though the whole outpost probably wouldn't hold that many. Just as I squatted behind a twelve by twelve support, a satchel charge came in the door, and all I remember is a big flash of white light. I had put all of my eggs in one basket and they blew up my basket.

I don't know how long we were buried. It was dusk when we were hit, and dark, I think, when the Chinese dug us out. I was blinded at the time and could only see blurs of light. I could not move. The twelve by twelve was across my chest, and one was across my helmet. It was probably an hour after I woke up that the Chinese started digging us out. I could feel arms and legs all around, but no one was moving or crying out. When they did get me out of the bunker—what was left of it—they put a bandage around my eyes. I didn't know if it was a blindfold or a bandage. And they started pushing and shoving me.

There was still lots of artillery all around. We went approximately three hundred yards and went into a tunnel. Then I realized they had probably tunneled up through our outwire.[2] The tunnel was about four feet tall and three feet wide. I was tripping all over bodies in the tunnel; I don't know if they were Chinese or Americans. The tunnel was probably a thousand yards long. When we came out, we were in a large trench. That was a big trench!

They put me in a truck with four or five wounded Marines or GIs, and we were driven for a long way to a small area with several huts. We were put in this place for two to three days. No food or water. Cold as it could be. One Marine, Sammy Armstrong, probably eighteen years old, had a bad arm wound. I thought he was really bleeding one night; I couldn't see. It was dark; I still had my bandage on. When I checked him, I could smell gangrene. I tried to rouse the guards and they hit me. But they took Sammy off, and when I saw him during the exchange of prisoners of war, he was absent an arm but otherwise in good shape.

We walked for approximately one day and came across a wounded Army man from West Virginia. He could not walk; I could not see, so we made a good pair. I carried him on my back and he told me where to walk. We came to what was later found to be an old abandoned gold mine. I think they called it Camp No. 10, way up in the mountains. Another Geronimo gave me a bath and washed my clothes in a stream. About ten of us were in a small room.

My presence really confused the Chinese. I was in Marine clothes with Navy insignias on my shirt. I think they thought I was a forward observer for the artillery or the big ships sitting out there shelling them all the time. So I was in isolation for a long time. My isolation "domain" was a hole in the ground five and a half feet long, three feet wide, and four feet deep with several two-by-four boards about one inch apart covering the opening. This turned out to be the camp's latrine. My uniform at that time was a T-shirt, fatigue pants, no shoes or socks. This was where they retrieved me for the firing squads.

Food was a very small handful of rice daily. Then I had fifteen to sixteen straight days of fake firing squads. They would go through "ready, aim, fire," then click. At that time, I was hoping they would kill me. That takes a lot out of you. Once or twice they'd send a live round close to my head into the rock wall behind me to get my attention.

It was cold. My feet, toes, and fingers were black, but I never lost any toes, fingers, nose, or ears. Even today, when my feet get cold, everything tingles and hurts. The song "Hand on My Shoulder" was so evident and alive then, long before it was written.

The camp was high in the mountains so no barbed wire could be used. They would hit our ankles with rifle butts, which caused so much swelling we could not walk very far. There was a young Marine with a bad wound in our camp, who had a tattoo of an American flag over his right deltoid muscle. There was a tear on his shirt over the tattoo. He would unveil that flag to everyone—a beautiful site. We even said the Pledge of Allegiance to our flag. The Chinese beat us every time they caught us. Finally they took him with me to the firing squad routine, tied his hands behind him, put him on his knees, put a gun to the base of his skull, and killed him three feet from me. God rest his soul!

Name, rank, and serial number didn't seem to impress them. They had never heard of the Geneva Convention. For me, the brainwashing really started then. After a few rifle butts to the head and body, I told them I was from Mississippi, had a mother, father, and two brothers. I was accused of germ warfare. I didn't know what on earth they were talking about. Then the bad cop/good cop routine started. After about four days of no sleep, being kicked and hit with rifles, and so forth, you learn to fake unconsciousness after the first rifle butt to your head or ribs, like Pavlov's dogs.

We had a Chinese interrogator who graduated from the University of Illinois, or Chicago, and had a masters in sociology. Wow! We named him "Blood on Hands" because he kept reminding us we had Chinese blood on our hands. He informed us that we had killed 5,000 Chinese, the first indication that we had done well. He kept trying to get me to sign the germ warfare papers, inform him of our battle strength and so forth, plus tell him which division we were from. Once again, I think they thought I was a forward observer for artillery strikes.

One time after a firing squad, he told me that the International Red Cross had informed him that my mother, father, and brother were killed in a car wreck. I was wondering how the IRC [International Committee of the Red Cross] knew I was there. I asked him about my sister. He said she was also killed. I had no sister. By that time, I was pretty mad. I informed him that he was lying. I had no sister. He hit me and called in some guards. They held me down and pulled my fingernail from the right ring finger with pliers. It had been injured earlier. It never grew back. It is a constant, daily reminder to me of my captivity. Nothing can be done to correct the nail bed.

On what I suppose was Easter, they gave all of us a dyed egg. Later on, we learned from one of the cooks, an Australian, that Stalin had died. I guess we thought it was like the old Wild West. If the Indian chief were killed, the Indians would stop fighting. We were so happy in a quiet way. We found out there were some Cuban POWs there also. We had two Australians in our hut; one was a cook.

By the grace of God, I had a tube of ophthalmic ointment in my top pocket which I kept putting in my right eye. Finally the eyesight on the left returned. The wounds on my leg, knee, and shoulder were healing. The Australian cook kept me supplied with some boiling water, and I kept pouring it on all of my wounds to remove the exudate. Thank God for the 23rd Psalm in my Bible. My mother had given me one with a steel case cover inscribed with "May this keep you safe from harm."

One day they loaded us on a truck and we headed out. There were no bombing runs by allied planes or artillery. We noticed in the morning that the sun was on our left which meant we were headed south. Still no noise of war going on. Were we really headed south? Still no noise of war going on.

We arrived in Kaesong and were held in an old Buddhist temple full of artillery and machine gun holes. I met other POWs. We were given clean bandages, Chinese clothing, and tennis shoes, none of which fit. We were told we were part of "Operation Little Switch," an exchange of sick and wounded POWs. Peace talks at Panmunjom were going on at that time.

I was there for three or four days before my name was called. I guess they tried to soften us up a little bit. We saw a Korean opera one day, a Chinese opera the next day, a real culture shock. There was some exchange of experiences and stories among other POWs. Most were dumbfounded, depressed, and there was not much talking. Most had very hollow looking faces. This is where I ran across Sammy Armstrong again. Glad he made it, but sorry he lost his arm. He was so young. Of course, I was an old twenty-year-old myself.

My name was finally called. I was loaded on the truck and headed for Panmunjom. We all cheered and cried when we saw the first Americans in uniform. We were taken to Freedom Village. The first nurse I saw was a lieutenant in the Army. I can't remember her name, but boy, was she beautiful. She took the bandage from my right eye and almost passed out. I realized then that it must be pretty bad. I ran into a corpsman, Bobby, from Tennessee. I can't remember his [last] name, but we were in corps school together. He told me about the high casualty rate on Reno, Vegas, and Carson. Woody and most others were killed. They already had a memorial service for me.

Notes
[1]"Operation Little Switch," the agreement negotiated at Panmunjom, called for 450 South Korean and 150 non-Korean prisoners to be sent south, and 700 Chinese and 5,100 North Koreans to go north.

[2]Barbed wire placed out front of the Marine positions.

12

Healing

*T*he terrible consequences of war had to be dealt with. Bullets, exploding mines, shells, and mortar and grenade fragments caused the trauma, tearing into flesh, ripping limbs apart, puncturing vital organs, stomachs and intestines, and inflicting disfiguring burns. For the lucky ones, aid was nearby—a hospital corpsman or a physician. They knew what to do. Fighting shock and hemorrhage were their first priorities. With battle dressings, tourniquets, and hemostats, they stemmed the bleeding. They splinted fractures, administered morphine, and perhaps began intravenous plasma, serum albumin, or even whole blood to counteract shock. Sometimes the caregivers performed these treatments while under fire. More often, corpsmen's ministrations occurred at an aid station dug into the reverse slope of a hill or in an aid tent close to the front.

First by jeep or ambulance, then by helicopter, the patient was evacuated to a medical company, a nearby MASH, or a hospital ship where surgeons did what they could. The seriously injured may have continued their long journey through Naval Hospital Yokosuka, Japan, where they received more definitive care before flying on to Tripler Army Hospital in Hawaii, a way station back to the mainland. Navy policy provided for convalescence at a military hospital near their homes, and most patients took that option.

Some patients required multiple surgeries to rebuild missing jaws and faces or to make hands without fingers useful once again. Indeed, amputees were in a special category. Healing stumps required monitoring to prevent infection. Prostheses made of wood, plastic, and leather needed to be custom-made and fitted to the patient. And then the real work began—learning to walk with an artificial leg or lift a glass with a prosthetic arm, which was manipulated by cables and pulleys and controlled by the wearer's muscles.

These were the physical aspects of convalescence. Most of the wounded, scarcely out of their teens, were resilient and up to the physical task. Psychological recovery would be more difficult to measure. For many, the very traumatic moment of their injury would be relived again and again in vivid nightmares and manifested with physical symptoms, such as sweats, panic attacks, and the shakes. Fourth of July celebrations or a car backfiring would send a veteran diving for cover. More than a few would turn to alcohol. The toll on marriages and family life will never be known.

Because the services of disabled Marines and sailors were no longer needed, they were discharged as soon as they were physically capable of leaving the hospital or being transferred to Veterans Administration hospitals for further care. All faced an uncertain future.

* * *

The Smell of Cordite

Peter Bingheimer was a corporal attached to Company H, 3rd Battalion, 7th Marines, at a place called "Outpost Frisco" near the 38th Parallel. The physical wounds he suffered at this outpost in a terrible nighttime firefight are still visible— a mangled left hand and an x-ray he often carries around as a memento. The x-ray shows the image of a communist burp-gun slug still nestling beside one of his vertebrae. Although he has adjusted to these injuries, treatment for his post-traumatic stress disorder (PTSD) is ongoing. The frightening dreams of what happened that night so long ago are less frequent now but occasionally reoccur. "All of a sudden, I'll wake up at night and smell the cordite. It's burned into my brain and I can't get rid of it."

I was assigned to a company in the 7th Marines and got shot at every day until I left there in October of 1952. After they sat down to talk truce, there was nothing but artillery fire, mortars, and sniper fire. The Chinese would think nothing about dropping a couple of thousand rounds on top of us every day and every night.

We were three miles from Panmunjom, at a very important main outpost called the "Hook." It was heavily defended because it was the invasion route from the north into Seoul. We had outposts about a thousand yards in front of it. And every two days they would change the personnel on those outposts because men were getting killed and wounded so fast.

I ended up replacing some men in an outpost called "Outpost Frisco," about two thousand yards in front of the Hook. It was constantly being probed and blasted with artillery. The outpost was in control of UN forces, and the object of the Chinese and us was to try and get a prisoner. But all we ended up doing was killing each other. There were minefields and booby traps of all kinds. It was high anxiety, believe me.

October 6th is the Chinese Moon Festival, and they decided to celebrate by taking our outpost. All the outposts along the line were attacked that night. I can remember everything and that's one of my problems. Around nine it was pitch-black. The moon didn't come out until two in the morning or so. All of a sudden, they must have thrown about a thousand rounds of artillery on top of us. Then they came at us screaming. We figured there were about three hundred of them; there were twenty-nine of us on the hill at the time. Their artillery smashed a lot of the barbed wire and they got through. From then on it was unbelievable. It was hand-to-hand fighting, blasting away at everybody. Everywhere you looked there were the killed and wounded. It was madness! They were throwing concussion grenades into our trench line. I grabbed two grenades and threw them back. The third one went off in my hand and knocked me back quite a ways.

Two fingers and the tip of another were blown off. I couldn't stop to monkey with them. And I couldn't use my M1 because the artillery bombardment had loaded it with so much dirt that it wouldn't function. I had to find another weapon so I grabbed a burp gun from one of the dead Chinese and started spraying them, and they started going down.

That burp gun was the only thing I had. That and anything I could pick up and throw at them. One guy stepped on my head and all over me. Another time I looked up and there was a Chinese about thirty feet down the line who opened up and hit me right in the chest with his burp gun, but my flak jacket stopped any of the slugs from penetrating. I still have five marks on my ribs where they were cracked.

This went on for about twenty-five minutes or so. We all ended up in a bunker trying to protect ourselves. When you were overrun like that, and if you had a radio, you could communicate back to the main line. We had a system called "box us in." They would throw 105s, 155s, and 8-inch shells on top of the hill. The shells had proximity fuses so they would explode in the air. We were in that bunker hunkered down, and they just threw hundreds and hundreds of rounds of this stuff on top of us. It was very effective in chopping up the Chinese. It just made spaghetti of them.

But that night the Chinese still came. One of them entered our bunker and sprayed us. That's where I got that slug in my back. It's a 7.62mm burp gun slug and it's been in my back since October 6, 1952. I got eleven different wounds from eleven different missiles, and there are some still in there. We also counted fifty-two pieces of shrapnel besides that.

Dawn came. The Chinese got a few prisoners, and they started withdrawing to the rear. When it got a little bit lighter, our F4U Corsairs came over the outpost and started strafing it. And then when the sun came, there was an eerie quiet. Before long, we heard voices talking in English in the background. They were people from Item Company. Somebody dragged me out of there and managed to get me to the reverse side of the next hill. From then on it was a trip to a helicopter. They took me to another place and transferred me to a bigger helicopter, which flew me to the USS *Repose* out in Inchon Harbor. I'll never forget what happened when they transferred me from the helicopter stretcher to the *Repose* stretcher. I apparently had a fragmentation grenade in my back pocket and it fell out onto the deck. Everybody scattered. Someone finally picked it up and threw it in the ocean.

I was exhausted. I remember waking up and finding myself in a smaller ward with a bunch of Korean marines and seeing nothing but slanted eyes; I thought I was a prisoner of war. I had an operation on my hand that day, and after four days, we sailed to Yokosuka and I went to the naval hospital there. Eventually, I was air-evaced to Midway, then to Tripler General in Hawaii, Oak Knoll [Naval Hospital Oakland] in Oakland, California, Andrews Air Force Base in Maryland, and then Bethesda.

There they performed a few operations on my hand to see if they could restructure it and offer me a better grip. And they worked on my eardrums. Both of them were blown out and I could hardly hear anything. They fixed one and the other I had taken care of when I got out of the Marines. They also took the bigger fragments out of my back and neck. There's still that slug in my third lumbar, but it doesn't bother me except when I think about it. It's a precarious situation. I don't know what would happen to me if I ever got hit hard back there. I might end up a paraplegic.

The people in the maxillofacial division in the dental clinic made me a cosmetic hand. They created a set of fingers that I could put over my hand so it would look like I hadn't lost any fingers. I still have it today. It was an experiment to see what could be done.

I was medically discharged on April 30, 1953, and took the bus home to Buffalo where I looked around and tried to readjust. I had a tough time. I went to the VA Hospital in Buffalo for about five months where they did a couple of more operations on my hand. Then I packed up and went to LA for a year and lived with a friend of mine. I got more therapy treatments on my hand at the Wadsworth VA Medical Center [Los Angeles].

I had a bunch of jobs and then got into alcohol bad because I didn't know what I was suffering from. I've never been able to utilize my potential because of the anxiety problem. Then I began having bad dreams about being in that bunker with the Chinese running around. Even though the dream is more infrequent now, I can talk about it.

I don't have a rigorous schedule. I bowl and get out and meet people. I go to PTSD meetings at the Vet's hospital in Batavia, New York.

My PTSD group has changed my life. I was almost a recluse all those years. There are still some fellas who are in bad shape, all Korean veterans. One hasn't been out of his house for fourteen months. He used to come to meetings but doesn't anymore. There's another guy who goes out in the woods in the middle of winter for three or four days. Then there's another guy who has two houses and a family. He lives in one house by himself and only goes to see his family at dinner time. He stands by the other house as though he's on watch on the frontline over in Korea.

Since 1991, I've been on a drug called clonazepam. It's a combination of an antispasmatic for the shakes—a muscle relaxer and a mild tranquilizer. It's a miracle drug for me. For the twenty years after I got home, I wouldn't go up in an airplane. After I got on that stuff, I flew down to Washington for the groundbreaking ceremony of the Korean Memorial in June of 1992. And the next year I flew all the way to Korea. I thought I could put a little closure on things by going to Korea but there's no such thing as "closure."

* * *

"All I Wanted Was a Chance"

Hospital corpsman Dan Skiles had just turned twenty in 1952. Recently stationed at Naval Hospital Oakland, California, he received orders to the Fleet Marine Force and then graduated from Field Medical training. Two weeks later he left his new bride and joined a draft of five thousand Marines aboard a crowded transport for Korea.

From then on, his experiences were similar to other Navy corpsmen helping to hold the line among the contested hills along the 38th Parallel. After a brief orientation, he was assigned to Company G, 3rd Battalion, 1st Marines, as one of two corpsmen in his platoon and obtained his "baptism of fire right off the bat."

I had no sooner joined the company when I was told to go on a night patrol. I knew no one. I went out with one of the squads and up a hill. It was my first introduction to a combat line outfit. I was scared to death. I had no idea where I was, who the old-timers were, or anything. As a corpsman, you had to be known and you had to know your men. If you didn't, you were going to get killed real quick.

I was walking along the trench line and being sniped at all morning and didn't even know it. "Gee, they've got some funny sounding bugs here." Then one bullet came pretty close to my head, and I suddenly realized that some idiot over there was shooting at me. He wasn't a very good shot or he would have gotten me very easily.

We were in and out of striking distance of the 38th [Parallel]. We pulled one week of guard duty on two of the bridges across the Imjin and that was like "R & R," rest and recuperation. They used to call it "I & I," intercourse and intoxication—that sort of stuff. I never got to pull any legitimate R & R. I wasn't there that long. But you'd get to the point where you'd start pushing your luck. I didn't sleep at night after the second month. That's when all the crap happened—at night.

I got hit at 11:30 at night on the 31st of August 1952. I had been pushing my luck. We were a half mile off Freedom Road out on a question mark-shaped point or hill surrounded by the enemy. They could shoot at us but there were certain areas where we couldn't shoot back because of the peace talks and no-fire zones.

We had one reinforced company of Marines and were seven and a half miles out in front of our Main Line of Resistance. If the peace talks fell through, our job was to go into Panmunjom, rescue the negotiators, and get them back to our main line.

We were almost right in the village of Panmunjom—their main line—at a place called Outpost Number 2. It was like the Santa Ana Freeway with traffic going in two different directions—trucks, tanks, everything. They moved mostly at night but you could hear and identify them by the sound. One of our guys was killed, and I had to go out several hundred yards in front of the lines to pick him up.

That night we were under attack and getting a lot of flak from outside our command post, which was well camouflaged. My platoon sergeant, Cornelius Harney, had been wounded. I took his boots and clothes away from him [to keep him from returning to action]. I and a new corpsman—a third class—were taking care of some casualties—nothing major—and planned on evacuating all of them.

I then went out to check the lines and was just heading back to the CP [command post] bunker. As I got close to my own bunker, there was Harney. He had gotten his boots and his pants back. I told him to come into my bunker so I could reinforce his bandages before he dropped. Just as I was going to slap him with a syrette of morphine, the crap started up again. The enemy was less than a hundred yards away. You could hear the mortars leave the tube. They'd go almost straight up and then come down.

So out went Harney again and all I could do was follow him. Suddenly it quieted down and I said, "OK, let's get back to our CP." So he headed back with me following him. That's when I heard three of those damn things leave the tube. I pulled him down in the trench, me on top of him, and held him down. One mortar round went to the left, one went to the right, and the other one landed right in my face, wounding me in all four limbs and the face. I was never knocked unconscious, but they had to get a pick and shovel to get Harney up. I was wearing a flak jacket and that's the only reason I'm alive.

Willy Workman, a corpsman who was with another platoon, was real close and got me into a bunker. Even though he got me pretty well patched up and started me on serum albumin— we weren't using plasma—I was going into shock very quickly so they slapped me with some morphine. It was almost like magic. And was I thirsty! They wet a bandage and let me suck on it and the thirst went away.

Because it was night, they couldn't get a 'copter in so they carried me off the hill back to Freedom Road, a good half mile away. After getting me aboard a jeep, we went seven and a half miles over that gravel road back to our company med where they reinforced my bandages and started me on whole blood.

After they were able to get a 'copter in, they put me in a basket on the outside and flew me back to Easy Med where they took some x-rays, reinforced the bandages, and gave me some more blood. They quickly decided I was in too bad a shape so they put me inside another 'copter, underneath the pilot, a Marine captain. He kept looking at me—concerned. He seemed like a nice guy so I decided to put him at ease by smiling at him. But I must have moved because blood spurted out of my shoulder. I thought the guy was going to crack up the 'copter so I decided that I had better not look at him anymore.

We landed on the flight deck of the USS *Repose,* and I was admitted into surgery at 9:10 A.M. on the first of September. I was still conscious from the time I was wounded until I went into surgery.

I don't remember anything after that for quite a while, and I don't know how long I was in a coma. I lost track of time. I now know that they had me up on the SOQ [sick officers' quarters] in a private room. I was having a helluva nightmare when I finally snapped out of it and came to. A Navy nurse was there, a jaygee named Kim. She was Japanese and we called her "Kimmie." The first thing I could see was my stump—the right leg. I could still feel my left arm so I didn't know that it was also missing. Kimmie said, "Danny, what's wrong?"

"My goddamn leg's gone," I said. "Can't you see it, you stupid bitch?"

She immediately broke down in tears, and that ended any bitterness I had. A couple of days later I was moved out to the regular orthopedic ward. And while I was there, Chuck Callahan, a friend of mine, walked in still wearing fatigues. Well, they kept Chuck with me from that point on. It was good therapy.

I first asked Chuck to get a wheelchair and take me up to SOQ where I apologized to Kim. I felt a lot better. It was something I had to do. Once in a while after that, she'd drop in and give me a big hug and kiss. The medical skipper on the ship would also come down and make my rack. He even gave me a shot of his private booze.

By that time, I had gotten back to being a corpsman again which meant I wasn't shocked about myself and my own body. I knew I was screwed up. I just didn't know how bad.

Every day they'd apply an elastic adhesive gauze to the leg stump and soak it with tincture of benzoin to keep the wound from dehydrating. It's kind of like putting Cosmoline on human beings but a lot stickier. There was a canopy over the leg while they were doing all this and changing the dressing so I couldn't see what was going on. I wanted to see my leg but they wouldn't let me.

One day a doctor asked if I minded if he took some pictures and I told him, "I sure as hell do."

"May I ask why?" he said.

"If I can't look at my own body, why should I allow you to take pictures of it?"

"If you could see, would you let me take pictures?"

I said, "Sure. Fair is fair."

So they finally took the canopy down, and I saw they had done a guillotine amputation—just a straight chop-off above the knee about midthigh.

From the *Repose*, I went to Inchon and then by ambulance rail to Kimpo Airfield. There I boarded a big Globemaster [C-124] with some other patients and flew to Japan. Navy ambulances then took us to Yokosuka Naval Hospital.

The next morning a Navy captain came by to check up on one of his patients. I knew him from my first duty station at Camp Pendleton. His name was Dr. [William] Cantrell. He didn't recognize me until he looked at my chart. Then he said, "What the hell happened to you?"

When I told him, he asked what they were going to do with me. I explained that we were supposed to fly out of there that morning. He said, "You don't want to go home looking like this, do you?"

"I don't even know if I wanna go home," I replied.

"Don't let them take you," he said. The *Haven* will be leaving here in about a week. They've got a bunch of good surgeons on that boat and we can get you in pretty good shape before you get home."

So I went aboard the USS *Haven* and we headed stateside. My buddy Chuck was still with me.

My two favorite surgeons were Dr. Hyatt and Dr. O'Dell. Several times they took me to Ear, Nose, and Throat and took the scabs off my eardrums; both were perforated. I also went to surgery two or three times before we got to Pearl Harbor. They did a revision on my leg by taking off a little more bone to effectively close the wound.

We got back to the States on October 13th and sailed under the Golden Gate. And for the first time, I was able to brush my own teeth by putting a toothbrush in the ace bandage on my hand. The minute we came under the Golden Gate Bridge, I was automatically back in the Navy. Up to that point, the Marines had been paying me and I had been dressed as a Marine. The Navy sent photographers aboard and that's when the famous picture was taken of me sitting on the edge of my bunk.

I was carried from the ship, put aboard a bus ambulance, taken to Oak Knoll, and placed in an overflow ward. The next day they moved us to the amputee ward where we got acquainted with a lot of other fellas. We had two wards devoted to amputees, and there were a lot of amputees at that time in Wards A and B.

My first night back I woke up about four o'clock in the morning and noticed someone near my bed. It was "Cats" Murphy, another nurse I had known when I was at Oakland before going to Korea. And she was crying—crying about me. You get pretty close to these people.

There was another nurse, Sarah Griffin, a leg amputee. She had lost her leg in Cuba falling off a cliff.

My first arm and leg prostheses were made there at Oak Knoll. The arm was the easiest to make. The only thing they had to do was hook up the pulleys and attach the bulkhead. The leg was something else. At the time, they made the leg from a block of elm. They finished it by covering it with rawhide and then painting it. The knee was like a hinge. The foot was wood with a soft pad on it. The ankle was a cable that [Dr. Thomas] Canty had designed with a bolt swaged onto the end of it so that you could snug it down where the tibia and fibula would be at the bottom of the ankle. He had a machine to test it at the speed of walking and ran it twenty-four hours a day to see how long this bolt would last. It was quite a thing in its day.

The bulkhead was made of leather at that time. Some legs were made of aluminum and/or sheet metal and covered with leather. They didn't have the total contact bucket at that time. It took time to develop these things because they were all done with hand tools and were quite involved. They were also nasty and hard to clean. The buckets would crack; you had to be careful you didn't drop it over a hard surface. I've always worn a suction socket.

I talked Dr. Canty into letting me take my leg home for Christmas. The arm wasn't difficult to handle but the leg required a lot of physical rehabilitation— walking, training, etc. He told me I could go home with the leg but not to try to walk on it, fearing I would get hurt. I went home and put the leg on anyway and it worked fine.

Having worked as a neuropsychiatric technician, I knew that whatever you do, the end result is going to be up to you. I didn't have the time. I had a wife, a family. I didn't have the luxury of spending too much time in the hospital. When I was coming back on the ship with Dr. Hyatt and Dr. O'Dell, they told me not to expect very much. I told them that all I wanted was a chance. And I got a chance. And when I get a chance, I make the most of it. It's that simple.

And I lost all the bitterness. Don't get me wrong. There have been times. But I learned to laugh at myself and once you learn to do this, you're OK. I knew enough about life to realize that if anything was going to come of it, I'd have to help myself a lot. I also had a lot of support. The main thing was that my wife stayed with me. A lot of guys didn't have that good luck.

When I first got back, life took a little getting used to. My wife had to get used to living with a cripple, so to speak. Actually, I think the only time I was crippled was when I was completely helpless and couldn't use my hand. But other than that, I've never been crippled. Even in my dreams I'm not an amputee. So, mentally, I've never accepted that I'm not a complete person. It might take me awhile longer and I may cuss a lot, but I get it done.

* * *

Nurse Amputee

One of Dan Skiles's caregivers was Sarah Griffin Chapman. The Georgia native graduated from nursing school during World War II, joined the Navy in 1944, and ended up in North Africa as the war in Europe was winding down. After serving at Naval Hospital Bainbridge, Maryland, she drew an assignment at Naval Hospital Guantanamo Bay, Cuba. One day while on a picnic, she fell from a cliff, fracturing the tibia of her left leg and breaking her right foot and ankle. Because the medical care she received was inadequate, she developed gangrene. Her left leg had to be amputated below the knee, ending her young career in the Navy Nurse Corps. When the Korean War broke out, her status changed once again.

When the Korean War came along, I wanted to go back on active duty, but I got a letter telling me I couldn't be assigned to special duty. Special duty meant that I could not be transferred from station to station. So I was very unhappy. I then wrote to BUPERS [Bureau of Personnel], but they still told me I couldn't come back into the Navy. But then they began getting all the amputees, and I assume that Dr. Canty, who had operated on me and fitted my prosthesis, talked to Rear Adm. [Clifford] Swanson, who was surgeon general of the Navy at that time. Soon I got a reply from Swanson asking me if I would come back on active duty and work with the amputees. I don't have his letter to me but I have the letter I wrote back to him. It says: "Since you think that I could render a valuable service to the Navy and to my country in rehabilitation of the amputees in the naval hospital, Oakland, California, I would be happy to volunteer for active duty for this assignment." I then got my orders to return to active duty in October of 1950.

I was very excited. I loved the Navy and I wanted to be a part of it. Dr. Canty wanted me because he liked how hard I worked to become a good walker. And I *was* a good walker and he felt that if I worked with amputees I could be of value. So I worked with the amputees from October 1950 to January of '53.

At Oakland, we had a ward full of patients, both below-the-knee, above-the-knee, and quadruples. I just worked with them and told them that if they put their minds to it, they could walk again. And if they worked hard, they could accomplish what they wanted to and live a normal life. You know, all the things amputees can do now. They skate, ski, run, play baseball and other sports. It's just miraculous what amputees do.

My days were very challenging, sometimes very disappointing, and sometimes very rewarding. There were so many different personalities to work with each day. Some didn't want to walk and I had to be creative to get them to. I wasn't on the ward but worked in physical therapy. Once a week I went around with Dr. Canty, a nurse, and two physical therapists, Charlie Asbelle and Jack Bates, both civil service employees. Jack was also an above-the-knee amputee. We'd make rounds and Dr. Canty would talk to the patients. The patients would then come down to see me. I'd talk to them about working on their balance and working to strengthening their legs and muscles. I told them they would have pain but that they would just learn to live with it. I told them that if they walked properly and did the things they needed to do like balancing and building up their muscles in the remaining leg and arms, why, they wouldn't have any problems.

We worked with the patients for two hours in the morning and two hours in the afternoon. In physiotherapy, which we called the walking clinic, Charlie Asbelle and Jack Bates guided me since I wasn't a physical therapist.

I generally worked with a group of about fifteen patients. They were all different. Some you didn't push. Some were gung ho. We saw patients all day long from eight o'clock in the morning until four o'clock in the afternoon. And they were mostly young men—eighteen, nineteen, twenty, twenty-one years old.

People who have a good muscle can wear a suction cup prosthesis. I didn't wear one of these. Because I was a patient for two years before my leg was amputated, I had lost all my muscle. I wound up with a stump shaped like a lightbulb with no muscle between the end of my stump and my knee. I don't have a lightbulb stump now but still can't wear a suction cup socket because of my circulation. But I walk all the time. Over the years, people sometimes noticed that I had a slight limp but, until 1990, no one knew I had a prosthesis unless they noticed the color of it. That year I fell and broke my left femur just above the knee. So now I have a limp and don't walk like I should. Nevertheless, I'm on my prosthesis twelve to fourteen hours a day. I don't do yard work anymore because my stump won't stand it. Everyone's afraid that I'll fall and hurt myself.

All these years later, I remember the times we had and the problems we faced. I think about many of my patients and wonder what happened to them. Sometimes I remember specific patients. I'd talk to a patient who was despondent and refused to walk. I was determined that he *was* going to walk. "I don't know why you want me to do this," he'd complain. "You don't know my pain. You have two legs and don't know how it is. You can't possibly know what I'm going through." At that point, I'd reach down and knock on my prosthesis. That would generally set them straight. From then on, they had no more excuses.

* * *

"If They Can Do It, Why Can't I?"

The memories of World War II were still fresh when Navy nurse Rosella Nesgis Asbelle began caring for the casualties of another war. As a Pearl Harbor survivor, she attended many victims of the Japanese attack. "It was really tragic," she recalls. "These kids were so young and so burned. I remember a radio blaring the song, 'I Don't Want to Set the World on Fire,' when some kid at the end of the ward yelled out, 'Lady, you're too late. It's done been set.'"

After the war, Lt. Nesgis attended the Boston School of Occupational Therapy, and was then assigned to Naval Hospital Mare Island, California, where she worked with amputees. When that hospital closed and personnel were transferred to Naval Hospital Oakland, California, she took charge of the occupational therapy department in 1950.

In the physical therapy department, amputees were trained to use their leg prostheses. They had a very active walking program for the amputees. In the occupational therapy department we worked with arm amputees and trained them to use their prostheses through a variety of activities and crafts that required them to manipulate their prostheses. We had a woodworking shop, a leather shop, and ceramics. The patients could choose whatever they wanted and often did several activities. They made little birdcages and small furniture like chairs, footstools, and other things. In the leather department they made wallets, women's purses, belts. In the ceramics department we had forms they could pour clay into. Some would do free-form and make whatever they wanted. We also had four or five looms and patients could make rugs.

The typical arm prosthesis was made out of metal with cables that attached to the shoulder muscles. Generally they had hooks. Later on they developed the hand. But the hand wasn't as convenient as the hook, which you could grasp anything with very quickly. It was just a two-pronged unit. The hand was a bit more difficult to control and harder to use.

I think the patients all did very well. They were intent on getting the most they could out of their rehabilitation and went for it. I can't remember any patient who didn't profit from the training. When they saw that others were doing OK, they'd say, "If he can do it, why can't I?" They were eager to learn as much as they could and get on with their lives.

* * *

"Bing" Crosby

Pfc. Harry Smart was a rifleman attached to Company E, 2nd Battalion, 7th Marines, when he received his wounds in the Nevada Cities fighting. As with many other injured Marines, he ended up on a Navy hospital ship. Following treatment there and in naval hospitals, he returned to duty, finishing his stint in the Marines as a drill instructor. For the next forty-eight years, he looked for "Bing," the Navy nurse who had intervened to save his leg.

We had just come off line from Hill 229, which was overlooking Panmunjom where the peace talks were going on. It seemed like just a few days when the Chinese and North Koreans decided to make a push down through the valley. At the front of the valley were the Nevada Cities outposts of Reno, Vegas, and Carson. This was about the 25th of March 1952. In the wee small hours of the 28th, we were sent out to reinforce Vegas, which had been overrun, retaken, overrun, and retaken. It was back and forth. The fighting was some of the fiercest during the Korean War. During this five-day engagement, there were three Medals of Honor awarded, eleven Navy Crosses, and more Silver Stars and Bronze Stars and Purple Hearts than you would want to count.

We had been up on line and the incoming from both sides was landing on one hill. That was our side shelling, their side shelling. On the 29th of March at about 0230 my luck ran out and I got hit with, I'm guessing, an 80mm mortar. It hit my right upper chest, blowing out some ribs, fracturing my pelvis, blowing it open to the bone. The projectile went through the right side and came out my stomach. My right boot was blown completely off and left shrapnel on the inside of the ankle.

I was then evacuated from the hill shortly thereafter. On the way down I had seen the South Korean people; we called them "chiggy-bearers." They'd run up and down those hills. They never stumbled, never tripped. But when they got me on the stretcher, all four of them tripped, and we all went bucket over teakettle off the top of the hill.

So, in addition to the wounds, I now had all the rest of the aches and pains. They eventually got down there to me and got me back to the MLR [Main Line of Resistance]. My first stop was at one of the aid stations. At that time I thought my leg was gone. When they got me into the tent, they asked how I was doing. I said, "I'm doing just great, but my feet are cold." I remember them elevating my feet up over the potbellied stove. I guess that should have been an indication that I still had both feet.

They treated me there, put me on the outside of a small helicopter, and transported me to one of the major med units. There they worked on me again. Eventually they transported me inside a larger helicopter which was extremely warm. Again I lost consciousness.

I woke up, I don't know how many hours later, on what I realized was a hospital ship. As they were off-loading me, I recall a corpsman or a doctor asking me how I was doing. I was in pretty bad pain but replied, "I'm doing just fine. Would you like to dance?" He chuckled and I chuckled and that's all I remember until I woke up in the ward.

I was hit on the 29th of March and woke up somewhere around the 3rd, 4th, or 5th of April. When I woke up, they were loading me on a gurney. I said, "Where are we going?"

One of the corpsmen replied, "You're going back to surgery. We need to do some more work."

And I said, "What kind of work are we going to do?"

And he told me, "Well, your right leg is of no value, and they're going to have to amputate it."

I said, "You mean I still have it?"

"Yes."

"Well, if I still have it," I said, "then I'm going to keep it."

A discussion ensued. About that time a Navy nurse came by and asked what the problem was. They told her we were ready to go to surgery, that I had regained consciousness, and was objecting to what was happening because my right leg was still there and I didn't want it taken off.

She went through the legalese to make sure I was awake and that I knew who I was. In a few minutes she told the corpsmen to put me back in the bunk, that I was not going back to surgery. And they insisted, "But the doctor said…"

And she replied, "But I said he's not going to surgery!" The nurse was probably a lieutenant (j.g.) at that time, but she dug her heels in and that was that. She then took care of me for the next two or three weeks. She was always there when somebody needed somebody to hold his hand, and she always had time to stop and talk to the guys—the ones who had lost legs and arms. She was just incredible. I remember her professionalism and her caring. I knew her name was Crosby but never knew her first name until 2000.

From what I understand, my initial surgery on the ship lasted about ten hours. I was pretty well shot up. My pelvis was fractured in two places and totally exposed. The back of my leg on the upper thigh looked like a hickory stick with the knots and stuff on it. They said all the nerves had been damaged and would never function. But it has functioned now for about forty-eight years and I'm still fairly good. I have good and bad days but that's to be expected with longevity.

After about two weeks on the *Haven*, we sailed to Yokosuka and I continued my treatment at the naval hospital. After they had gotten me up and moving, I had therapy. The wound on my hip was open all the way to the bone. It was bad. Part of my treatment included the sitz bath. One day I was sitting down in the sitz bath when a nurse came by and said, "How long have you been in there?"

I said, "Four or five minutes."

"Well, it's time to get out." The drain was on the right side and this was where I had been hit. She reached down, pulled the stopper out, and I thought it was going to suck all my insides out. I began hollering and the corpsman came and got me up out of there.

Nevertheless, I had a good stay at Yokosuka. I have nothing but admiration and praise for the Navy medical people. They're why I'm still here. It was a good experience.

I flew from Yokosuka to Wake or Guam, and then on to Tripler, where I spent the night. From there I went to Travis Air Force Base in California, and then on to the naval hospital at Mare Island where I spent three to four weeks. In between some of this, I was still having surgeries getting the shrapnel out. They were trying to locate me close to where my mother was, which was New York City. Eventually I wound up at the naval hospital in St. Albans, New York. That's where I spent the rest of my time until I got out and returned to duty.

My leg wasn't real good but at least I was off the crutches and I didn't have a cane. I was moving pretty good. But the hip was still open and it stayed open for several years. I still have a hole in it.

Despite my injuries, the Marines found me fit for duty. I guess I was in good enough shape. I went through DI [drill instructor] school and was able to function. They told me that as time went on my leg would become worse and it has. I'm having more problems with it now. I'm on pretty heavy medication for pain but it's manageable.

About four or five years ago, the Military Order of the Purple Heart wanted to do a special issue of their magazine honoring medical personnel who took care of us. They solicited stories from veterans. I wrote a story about my situation and how the nurse they called "Bing" saved my leg. At that time no one had ever heard of her; I certainly didn't know where she was. I submitted the article and it got published. I think this was in '95 or '96. A few years later, I read an article about a Navy commander named Frances Omori who was soliciting articles about Navy nurses during the Korean War. I wrote her a note and in a few weeks got a questionnaire which I filled out and returned.

About two months later, the phone rang and the person asked for Sgt. Smart. I hadn't been Sgt. Smart in years. The voice on the other end said, "Harry? This is Cmdr. Omori. Are you sitting down? I think I've found Bing."

I was stunned and couldn't say a word—the fact that she had found someone I had been looking for for forty-eight years. She gave me Bing's address and we began corresponding.

While at a Korean War veterans' reunion in Virginia Beach, I called Bing and asked if I could visit her. So I left Virginia Beach and headed for Florida. On October 15, 2000, I rang her doorbell. I'm not very good with words but I can tell you that we hugged and cried. It was incredible to find this lady who had saved my leg and my life so many years ago. I had no idea I would ever see her again.

* * *
Bing's Story

Frances Omori told Harry that she had interviewed me and had my address. She then wrote me and asked if I would mind if she gave him my address. I wrote back to her and said I'd be pleased to talk with him. Harry wrote the nicest letter and asked if he could someday come to see me. But we didn't meet until about two years later. In 2000, he drove all the way down to Florida just to see me.

Oh, it was very emotional at first. We hugged and cried. It was very warm and touching. I still get emotional when I talk about it. I don't know where the feelings welled up from but they really were something. I was very, very moved. He made all those years in Korea worthwhile.

In April 2002, Nancy Crosby accompanied Harry Smart and several other veterans to South Korea where they were honored by the nation they had all helped to save.

* * *
Marines and Rescuers

It was a terrifying time for a patrol to be caught out in no-man's-land. The safety of darkness was brightening with the first rays of dawn that misty morning in October 1951. Sgt. John F. Fenwick Jr., already a decorated and hardened veteran of the Chosin Reservoir campaign, felt the hair on the back of his neck standing straight up. Their new and very inexperienced lieutenant had taken them within several feet of North Korean lines. Moments later, a shot rang out signaling the beginning of a savage firefight in which most of Fenwick's comrades perished. The exchange left him bleeding and near death when at least four machine gun bullets ripped through his body. As a hospital corpsman dragged him to safety, he, too, was severely wounded. Despite those injuries, the sailor did what every corpsman is trained to do—protect his patient, administer first aid, and see the wounded Marine safely to the rear.

The story does not end there. It took a skilled Navy surgeon many hours to repair the damage and put Sgt. Fenwick on the long road to recovery. He recalls that unforgettable time half a century ago when Navy medicine came to his rescue.

I'll never forget the date. It was 5 October '51. I was a machine gun squad leader in Co. A, 1st Battalion, 5th Marines. The captain called us in and told us he wanted a prisoner to interrogate. He told me I would be relieved in two days and then would probably be going home. He then said I didn't have to go on this patrol. We had a brand new green lieutenant who had only been with us two days. I figured

I had better go because he'd need some advice. A good officer will listen to his NCOs who had combat experience.

We were northeast of Inje, close enough to the ocean to have naval gunfire from the battleship *Missouri* supporting us. We went out before dawn. The lieutenant disobeyed orders and got us all fouled up. We ended up in the enemy lines. You could hear them talking and starting their cooking fires. It was scary as hell. We then pulled off that hill and instead of going right back to our lines and taking advantage of the heavy ground mist, the lieutenant said, "Let's try that other hill."

The platoon sergeant who outranked me kept telling him we had to get back to our lines. "You can't make a name for yourself out here because you're gonna get everybody killed," he said.

The mist burned off and we were exposed out there, almost like someone had turned on a light switch. Then one shot rang out. Lyons, a friend of mine, was at the point [up front] and got one right between the eyes. We were only fifty yards from some of their bunkers, maybe even closer than that.

We ran behind a nearby knoll but they continued to fire at us from two sides and the front. We got the machine gun set up on the knoll and began to answer fire. But it was like taking a motorcycle and running up against a tractor trailer. We had literally hundreds of them shooting at us. The whole platoon got shot to pieces. The lieutenant then called in supporting artillery and when they registered in, the shells landed right on top of us on that hill. I guess he fouled that up, too. Finally they corrected and the shells began landing on enemy lines.

By then, just about all of us were hit. Our machine gun was out of ammunition and was knocked out. I was the last guy alive on that knoll. I saw some of the enemy trying to work their way around our right and get behind the hill where all our wounded were. Our corpsman, Glen Snowden, was treating the wounded below. So I grabbed an M1 off the dead kid who was lying beside me, and I raised myself up to shoot at the infiltrators trying to outflank us. That's when I got it—four hits in the body—machine gun bullets. We were so close I could feel the muzzle blasts. It was a Russian light machine gun. When you were in Korea awhile, you could tell every weapon firing at you.

It's indescribable the way it felt. It was like being run over by a train. I was bent backwards. It turned out that two of the bullets grazed my spine. I could feel everything else except for my legs. It was horrible pain.

Doc Snowden came running up and grabbed me. He checked everyone else real quick but saw that everybody else up there was dead. He said, "I've gotcha; I'll get you out of here." As he started pulling me, the machine gun got him twice in his left shoulder and knocked him right down the hill. He scrambled right back up again. One arm was hanging down and useless, but he still grabbed me and got me out of the line of fire.

He began telling the unwounded rifleman how to dress guys' wounds. I had an artery severed on my left flank [side], and the exit wound in my back was the size of a fist. Apparently the bullets had hit my ammo belt and tumbled. Some hit my small intestine and I eventually lost eighteen feet of my small intestine, which is nothing. If they had hit my large intestine, that would have really been bad.

Snowden dragged me out of there with one hand. When I finally got back to our lines, I told the guys to write him up for a Silver Star, at least. He saved a lot of guys besides me. He grabbed a jacket off one of the dead Marines and rolled it up into a ball; he was all out of battle dressings. He then put it against that hole in my back and took another jacket and tied it around me real tight, like a compress, to stop the flow of blood. And that's what saved me. He had some morphine syrettes left, and told a BAR [Browning Automatic Rifle] man, [Cpl. Richard] Baiocchi, to give me some morphine. Baiocchi then said, "Here, I'll give you some morphine." He stuck the morphine syrette in my shoulder.

I was looking into his face and saying, "Thank you, pal" or something like that, and just then a machine gun burst hit him right in the jaw and sheared it off. His whole chin was gone! He also took six rounds between his wrist and elbow.

Unfortunately, I didn't get the morphine because as he got hit, the impact snapped the needle off while it was still in my arm. The pain was unbelievable. It was like someone had opened me up with a scalpel without any anesthetic and then filled up my insides with red hot embers.

I forgot to mention that when Doc Snowden grabbed me, two more bullets got me in my left upper arm. One was a graze and the other went through the flesh real quick.

After Snowden got through with me, two Marines grabbed each of my feet and dragged me face down back through the rice paddies. They were under such fire that they had to run, dragging me on my face through all that muck. It's a wonder I didn't drown.

When we got back a ways, they put me on a litter. I really thought I had died because when we got halfway back, I felt warm and peaceful. All the pain left me. While I lay face down on the stretcher, I saw a real bright orange, hazy light, but there was no pain. I remember thinking, "Thank God, it's all over."

Right about then there was an air strike on the enemy position and that pulled me out of it. It really made me feel good thinking that the ones who got me were getting fried with napalm.

When we got back to our own lines, I was still conscious. A helicopter landing pad had been dug out on the reverse slope of a hill. They didn't think I was going to make it. Only one chopper could be brought in there at a time, and there was only room for two wounded on each. There were so many wounded, they could only take the ones who had a chance of making it. Some of them went down the hill on stretchers.

A chief corpsman told one of the surgeons to look at me. I remember he had a big walrus moustache. "Sir, you had better look at this man. It looks like his color's still good."

The doctor then said, "Take one of them out of the basket and put him in."

It was just a plain chicken wire basket like you see on ships. There were no blankets or anything. They had just dumped me in the basket face down. The guy in the other basket was a rifleman from Texas. He had four bullet wounds stitched across his chest. He didn't make it. And he had three kids at home.

When we lifted off, I got a panoramic view of the whole hill we had been fighting for for so long. It was really something to see. I could see all the guys down below and the positions. I also saw blood splattering all over. I didn't realize it was my blood being splashed all over the place by the rotor blades. I had a severed artery. They had a compress on it but it was still bad.

They flew us back to Easy Med ["E" Medical Company]. I remember being very scared. They put me on a slanted wooden table and cut all my clothes off. Then they put a catheter in my penis. The surgeon's name was [Lt.(j.g.) Howard] Sirak. He and the other surgeon really put me at ease. And then with his finger he drew a line on my stomach and said they were going to make a small incision. That was no small incision. They ended up cracking me open—a laparotomy! Dr. Sirak later told me they put 837 sutures in me. Rather than making a colostomy, they kept snipping perforated small intestine off and re-sewing [the ends] together.

When I woke up, it was night. I only saw one Coleman lantern at one end of the tent. I was lying on the cot and felt all warm and sticky on one side. I had dysentery once and thought I had messed myself. I called a corpsman who came to me with the lantern. He said, "Don't worry, it's just blood." I had blood and plasma going in both feet and both arms—IVs. There was a Levin tube[1] coming out of my nose, another tube in my penis, and another coming from the exit wound in my back.

The next morning both surgeons came in. They told me they had to get me up on my feet. I said, "You've gotta be kidding me. I'm dyin' here. I can't feel my legs; I can't move."

He said, "When we got in there we found three vertebrae that were just grazed by the bullets and were fractured. But you have what they call spinal shock. The feeling will return. We can practically guarantee it."

But I was really worried I was going to be a paraplegic. But, for the grace of God, another eighth of an inch, I would have been. The bullets had tumbled their way through me. Then I got peritonitis real bad. I remember by the time I got to the hospital ship, I was getting 500cc's of penicillin a day. It could have been fragments of filthy clothing going through with the bullets or stuff from the rice paddy, and, of course, perforated intestines. I remember the day I got hit I hadn't had anything to eat, just a sip of water. The surgeon said that had I had food in my intestines, that probably would have been it. I wouldn't have survived.[2]

From there they sent us to the hospital ship—the *Consolation*. They put us in slings and hoisted us aboard. It looked great. It was snow-white—unbelievable! The ward was so clean and beautiful. I think it was even air conditioned. I didn't want to get in that bunk. It was so clean and I was so filthy. There was all the crud from the front plus blood caked all over me. I hadn't been in a bed in over a year. When they got me all cleaned up and in a bunk, gave me all my shots, and changed my dressings, the nurse, a lieutenant commander, said, "How would you like to have some ice cream?"

I couldn't believe it. I thought, I'll really fool her. So I said, "Yeah, I'd love to have some."

And she said, "What flavor?"

And knowing they wouldn't have it, I said, "Rocky fudge."

And then she said, "Coming right up, Sarge."

Then I completely lost it. I grabbed her hand and kissed it. Then I broke down crying. "You Navy nurses are really angels of mercy."

Sgt. Fenwick suffered six machine-gun bullet wounds. Two were through-and-through wounds of the left upper arm with no permanent bone, muscle, or nerve damage. Four were through-and-through wounds of the left flank, involving the small intestine, left pelvis, left iliac crest, and iliac joint, which was destroyed by direct trauma. A large exit wound in the lower left back was adherent to the lumbar spine with fractures of L-3, L-4, and L-5. The left artery was severed. Two of the gunshot wounds were "keyhole" rounds, which tumbled end over end, causing large muscle and tissue damage and loss in the lumbar spine region.

During the year Fenwick spent at the National Naval Medical Center recovering from his wounds, occupational therapy was one aspect of his treatment. He whiled away some of the time assembling ship models, but when a staff member gave him a drawing pad, a pen, and ink, a hidden talent emerged. His battlefield nightmares were transformed into sharp-edged drawings, photographically meticulous in every detail. The faces of his subjects reflected the "thousand-yard stare" of fighting men who had witnessed too much combat, known too little sleep, seen too much death. A bullet-riddled ambulance, its mutilated cargo strewn beside it, illustrates the "communist mercy" Fenwick had witnessed all too often in Korea. One drawing mirrors his own terrifying experience. A hospital corpsman tends to a fallen Marine as a plasma bottle drips its lifesaving contents into one of his veins. In the background, another man vigorously summons an overhead rescue helicopter.

For nearly half a century these drawings lay forgotten in a drawer until the artist showed them to a friend. Several were subsequently published in the May–June 2001 issue of Navy Medicine *magazine and are now in the collection of the National Naval Medical Center, Bethesda, Maryland.*

* * *

Glen C. Snowden, a World War II veteran, was no stranger to combat when he found himself in the same firefight that felled John Fenwick. Following Fenwick's interview, I located the former hospital corpsman and asked him what he recalled about saving his wounded comrade. Snowden was unaware his patient had survived his wounds. Having also relayed Fenwick's gratitude, I learned the next day that the two men had already spoken by phone, reuniting after almost fifty years.

I remember that day. I had to get him [Fenwick] up over the hill because he had slid down on the enemy side. If we stayed there, we'd both have been shot. So I grabbed him by the ankles and told him, "Put your arms on your stomach and hold them down real good." And then I said, "I'm gonna pull you up."

He said, "No. I don't think I can make it."

And I told him, "You're gonna make it because I'm going to start pullin' right now." I tied his hands together and put both my hands underneath his armpits as far as I could. Then I got his head up on my chest and started moving. I wanted his head up high where I could see whether he was breathing or not. You don't want [your patient] to bleed from the mouth. If they do, they can choke. And that's the way I pulled him back up. The only thing that stayed on the ground as I pulled him were his heels.

Then I was wounded myself. I was standing up at the wrong time—very stupid, but I wasn't bleeding. I plugged that up. I put a peg in it. I'd take a limb and kind of smooth it with my knife. Then I'd break it off. I'd make a couple of them and put them in my pocket. Then, if I got shot, I'd just stick one in the wound real fast, and it wouldn't bleed. You'd be surprised how that worked.

So I got him up there [on the backside of the hill], and the first thing I had to do was bandage him. I tore his shirt in the back where the bullets had come

out and patched him up there. I put a great big [battle dressing] on him and
tied it as tight as I could get it. And then I turned him over and patched up his
stomach. That's when the corpsmen started yelling that they had a vacant litter.
We grabbed him underneath the arms and put him on that litter and they took
off. I yelled, "Good-bye. You're goin' back to the States. I wish you all the
luck in the world. I know you're goin' to make it back, so take it easy." And
he waved at me.

I never found out what happened to him after he left. I called after I got back
down to the base, but they must already have taken him. I guess they put him
right on that hospital ship. As long as I was over in Korea, nobody would send
any information through on the radio telling me what happened to him. I guess I
probably saved quite a few lives over there, but I sure put everything in it when I
saved him.

* * *

*Cpl. Richard Baiocchi had taken over when Snowden, too weak from loss of
blood, could no longer help Fenwick. He instructed the Marine to give Fenwick a
shot of morphine and that's exactly what Baiocchi was doing when another burst
of fire from a machine gun sheared off his jaw and pierced his right shoulder and
left arm.*

I had never given anyone a shot of morphine before but there's a first time for
everything, I guess. Suddenly I was hit in the left arm, right shoulder, and my jaw.
I just couldn't comprehend what was going on. In fact, Glen [Snowden] got hit at
the same time. I remember him saying that he couldn't help me. He then told me
to run back and try to get to some South Koreans who were trying to help us out
with stretchers. All this time the enemy was shooting at us. They put me on a litter
and while I was lying there, the North Koreans were still shooting. The helicopter
finally came, and I very faintly remember them getting me in the basket on the
outside. Then they flew me back to the field hospital.

That was the last I remember. When I got to the field hospital that's where they
saved most of my face. I don't even know how long I stayed there in the field
hospital. I don't even remember if they sent me to a hospital ship. I could have
been on one but I don't remember. From there they flew me to Yokosuka, Japan. I
was there between thirty and sixty days. After I left Japan, I stopped off in Hawaii
at Tripler Army Hospital and stayed there for two or three days. From there they
flew me to Travis Air Force Base in California, and I was there for thirty days.
From there I made a couple of stops including Lackland Air Force Base and then
an Air Force base in Alabama. I think they just transferred me from one plane to
another. From there I flew to Andrews Air Force Base in Washington. They had an

ambulance waiting for me and they took me right to Bethesda. The next day they started my treatments.

I almost lost my left arm. They kept pulling bullets out of my arm even after I got to Bethesda. I think they took three of them out there. There were seven holes in my right shoulder. They worked on my arm there but they didn't do all that much with my jaw. That's why they transferred me to Philadelphia.

My jaw was almost off. That's why I took so long in the hospital with all these operations. They took a piece of bone out of my hip and grafted it to my jaw. Then I got an infection in my jaw from that operation, osteomyelitis. They had to reopen it and scrape the bone to get rid of the infection. The wires are still in there. My jaw was wired up for a long time and all I could eat were liquids. I was on that liquid diet for a couple of months. After they removed the wire, I went over to real soft foods.

Fortunately, my tongue wasn't affected, thank God, but my teeth were all knocked out, except four on top. In fact, those four are still intact. All my lower teeth were gone. I don't know how many operations the oral surgeons did but they did a good job. I remember one doctor came up to me and said, "We'll get you fixed up as good as we can but you know you'll never be the same as you were before." They made a special plate for inside my mouth with teeth attached to it. There was a commander at Philadelphia, an oral surgeon, who was really good. There was also a plastic surgeon there named Lt. [Richard] Oakey. They would operate on me and then would let me go home for thirty days. Then I'd go back and have another operation. Then they'd send me home for another thirty days. All told, I had fifteen operations between Bethesda and Philadelphia. This totaled almost two years—six months at Bethesda and eighteen months at Philadelphia.

I was discharged in 1953. The corpsmen and the nurses were fantastic. I was very pleased with the way they all treated me. Of course, I still have my scars there. But a lot of people have asked me where I was wounded, and they don't even notice that I was wounded in the jaw. I can't eat a tough steak or anything like that, and I have to chew my food a lot more than anyone else because of the special plate I have. But I can eat mostly everything.

I think they did a masterful job, but I feel the people in that field hospital were the ones who really saved most of my face. If it hadn't been for them, I don't know what would have happened.

* * *

Lt.(j.g.) Howard Sirak was on duty at Easy Med when they brought in all three men, two grievously wounded Marines and their corpsman with a lifeless arm dangling beside him. One of the Marines looked familiar, despite his missing jaw.

He said, "Hey Doc, don't you remember me? I'm Baiocchi." I remembered him. I had seen him about two weeks before for a minor shrapnel wound in the arm. And now here he was with his jaw shot off. All but the posterior parts of his mandible were pretty well broken up, even though there were still remnants of bone maybe the size of a half-dollar or quarter. You can't get hit with a machine gun bullet in the jaw without doing damage. And he had a hole in the floor of his mouth and his tongue was hanging out. There was also a lot of soft tissue damage, and it was obvious that he was going to require extensive plastic surgery. I didn't want him to lose any more through infection or loss of tissue so I put it back together as best I could. I sewed up the soft tissue in, around, and under his chin.

* * *

On 10 July 2001, the Marine whose insides were nearly blasted away, the buddy who lost his jaw trying to help him, and the Navy surgeon who attended them both were reunited in an emotional ceremony at the National Naval Medical Center in Bethesda, Maryland. The occasion was John Fenwick's donation of his long forgotten drawings to the hospital. After so many years of not knowing what became of these two patients, Dr. Howard Sirak was overjoyed to see both men whole again.

Notes

[1] A gastroduodenal catheter of sufficiently small diameter to permit insertion through the nasal passages.

[2] The presence of food would most likely have increased the chance of infection.

Postscript

At 10:00 A.M. on 27 July 1953, North Korean Lt. Gen. Nam Il and chief UN negotiator Gen. William Harrison signed the armistice, marking an end to the war and an uneasy truce that survives to this day. This event, however, had never been a foregone conclusion among those manning the trenches and bunkers along the 38th Parallel or patrolling the bomb line off the Korean coast.

"During the latter part of that cruise, we kept hearing rumors from Panmunjom about an armistice," recalled Navy doctor Lt. Clifford Roosa. "Several times peace seemed imminent and then the deal would fall apart. We were still having casualties. Our purpose became more unsure and I became jaded and discouraged. It was apparent that we weren't going to win this war, even if sometime there was going to be peace."

Roosa described the scene from the deck of the heavy cruiser USS *St. Paul* just before the truce went into effect at 10:00 P.M. on the 27th, twelve hours after the armistice papers had been signed: "It was remarkable. Because no one wanted the logistical problem of having to unload unspent ammunition when we got back, we let loose with all our guns. The entire peninsula seemed to be lit up. I don't know whether we had any specific targets; we were just getting rid of that damn ammunition. Just before midnight, we fired the last round. I understand that was the last round fired in the war. When it really happened, we didn't cheer or wave flags. We just went about our business."

A half-century has passed since that day, ample time to gain some perspective on the war. The mood of America in 1953 was simple and unmistakable. Like Dr. Roosa, Americans had grown weary of the conflict in Korea and discouraged over its victory-less conclusion. They, too, just went about their business, preferring to focus instead on other issues closer to home. The "forgotten war" was well on its way to becoming so.

The "fifties" were in full swing—Levittown, rock-and-roll, *I Love Lucy,* Dr. Salk's miracle vaccine, McCarthyism, the Cold War, and the backyard bomb shelter. For those who ruminated on the Korean War's significance, more than a few pointed out that without victory, the war had been a colossal mistake, certainly in terms of lives and treasure. What had been accomplished? The Korean peninsula was still divided, and now the United States was faced with the ominous conviction that the Free World's enemies—the Soviet Union and Red China—represented monolithic communism bent on world domination. True or not, these perceptions were Cold War realities for nearly the next forty years.

What has happened since 1953 provided more than a few surprises: the breakup of the Soviet Union; the winning of the Cold War; the opening of our adversaries' archives to the scrutiny of investigators and scholars; and the rewriting of history based on new documentation. And now with all this evidence and the benefit of hindsight, we can again reevaluate the Korean War.

When I began working on this book, I focused on one concern—the role of Navy medicine in the Korean War. The veterans I interviewed were either the caregivers or their patients, and my questions were medically related. What I could not predict was my subjects' willingness to go beyond the medical arena and share observations and opinions about the meaning of their war and how it had affected their lives since. Indeed, Dr. Howard Browne had said, "I don't know why they're calling it the 'forgotten war.' I can remember it as if it were yesterday."

Several of the veterans interviewed have even gone back to South Korea in recent years either to satisfy a lingering curiosity or to honor the memories of comrades who never came home. I ask these men and women one final question. Was all the blood and sacrifice worth it?

In June 2000, USS *Consolation* nurse Betty Gregorio Baker returned to Seoul as part of a special U.S. delegation to help celebrate the fiftieth anniversary of the war's beginning. The delegation included then-Secretary of Veterans Affairs Togo West and Congressman Charles Rangel, himself a Korean War veteran. The visit's climax took place at Seoul's Korean Memorial.

At the commemoration, Baker recalled some poignant and painful memories: "There were thousands of veterans wearing white hats to show they were veterans—South Korean veterans and veterans from each of the sixteen countries that had participated in the war. You looked out into the audience and knew that these were the men who were in the bunkers back then, without the proper clothing, and being shot at all the time. Many of their comrades were left for dead. I looked out at that sea of hats and was just so proud to be there with them."

Marine Gunnery Sgt. Garrison Gigg summed up what many of his comrades feel fifty years after the war ended in stalemate. "I took a trip to Korea two years ago and it was a hell of a release for me. I really felt good about it. When I saw the young kids running around fat and chubby-faced, it made me realize that what we did was really worthwhile. And when I look back then, I see the kids—skinny and dying in their mothers' arms. There was no food and we were feeding them whatever we had. Today, it's just amazing to see how their economy and their cities have grown. I feel good about things like that."

In April 2002, USS *Haven* nurse Nancy Crosby also returned to Korea, accompanied by several veterans, including Harry Smart, the Marine whose leg she saved from amputation aboard her hospital ship. They visited Inchon, Seoul, the demilitarized zone, the truce village of Panmunjom, and long-forgotten battlefields with unpronounceable names. The contrast between then and now was striking.

"Back then," Crosby recounted, "the only thing left standing in Seoul was the presidential palace and a Catholic church on a hill. There were a few hotels and buildings, but they were all pockmarked by bullets and shell fire. The rest of the city was blown away. What people sold then were ashtrays made from beer cans. The South Korean streets today are absolutely clean and spotless. There are flowers everywhere. Now, the cars are brand new. I didn't see any carts being pulled by oxen, which was all we saw fifty years ago. There are skyscraper apartment buildings, one right after the other from Seoul to Inchon.

"In Panmunjom the South Koreans showed us a satellite view of Korea at night, with the DMZ [demilitarized zone]and, below it—South Korea—all lit up. In North Korea there was just the occasional dot or dots that indicated electric lights. We knew that up there the people are still starving the way they were back then. The difference between the North and the South is night and day. Was it all worth it? Of course it was. The people of Korea are so appreciative of what we did. Wherever we went, they bent over backward and treated us royally."

Marine Sgt. Peter Bingheimer was also in for a surprise. "When we left Korea, the hills were just bare; there weren't any trees on them. They were blown to bits by artillery and napalm. Today it's just beautiful—forty years' growth of trees and bushes. I was amazed by how the people treated us. They treated me like a king. I was there six days and stayed in the finest hotels.

"The cities are all new because we blew them apart. Seoul has eleven million people and four and a half million automobiles. There are nineteen bridges over the Han River and seventy-story skyscrapers, and, of course, the ubiquitous McDonald's. Every day they took us on a tour of some part of the country. Everywhere the people just walked up to us, shook our hands, and said, 'Thank you for coming over.'

"I first went to Korea because my buddies had been killed and I wanted to go and avenge their deaths. We stopped the communists from taking over a democratic country. We did the right thing."

The veterans had answered my final question.

The Cast

MARILYN EWING AFFLECK left the Navy in 1956 to marry. In 1970, she returned to nursing as a civilian and retired in 1985. "When I came home from Korea, a fellow that had grown up near me said, 'You haven't been around in a long time. I thought you were dead.' I assured him that I was very much alive." She died in 2004.

ROSELLA NESGIS ASBELLE married Charles Asbelle, a physical therapist and colleague, while still working at Oakland Naval Hospital, and then resigned from the Nurse Corps with fifteen years of service. After raising a family, she became a real-estate broker. She makes her home in Oakland, California.

RICHARD BAIOCCHI, after his discharge from the Marine Corps, returned to his job at the Hershey Candy Company in Hershey, Pennsylvania. He is now retired and lives in Hershey.

PETER BINGHEIMER worked for the Internal Revenue Service, the U.S. Postal Service, and Customs Service following the war and retired from the Immigration and Naturalization Service after twenty-six years as an immigration officer. He lives in Tonawanda, New York.

JOEL BOONE, Medal of Honor recipient for World War I heroism, White House physician to three presidents, Third Fleet's Medical Officer during World War II, and the Navy surgeon general's eyes and ears following the Inchon landing, retired in 1950. He died in 1974.

HOWARD BROWNE's tour in Korea ended in January 1952. He retired from the Navy in 1967 after twenty-four years of service and lives in Williamsburg, Virginia.

SARAH GRIFFIN CHAPMAN was discharged from the Navy in 1953 and then worked part-time at St. Joseph's Hospital in Atlanta, Georgia, for nineteen years. She now makes her home in Tucker, Georgia.

NANCY "BING" CROSBY retired from the Navy as a commander in 1969 with twenty years of service. After teaching nursing at Seminole Community College in Annapolis, Maryland, for two years, she moved to Winter Springs, Florida, where she currently lives.

WILLIAM "BILL" DAVIS remained in the Navy, retiring as a commander in the Medical Service Corps. He divides his year between Florida and Wisconsin.

ROBERT DOBBIE made a career in the Navy and was assigned to many naval hospitals around the world. After training in cardiothoracic surgery, he became assistant chief of surgery at the National Naval Medical Center in Bethesda, Maryland. He retired as chief of surgery at Naval Hospital Oakland, California, after twenty-six years of active service. Dr. Dobbie then joined the faculty of the University of Tennessee in the Department of Surgery before becoming a medical director of Baxter Travenol Laboratories. He is now retired and lives in Lincolnshire, Illinois.

LURA JANE EMERY retired from the Navy as a commander after nearly twenty-seven years of service. She makes her home in Lancaster, Pennsylvania.

WAYNE ERDBRINK did a short deployment with another squadron after his wartime cruise on *Antietam* flying patrols out of Kwajalein before and after the first H-bomb testing in the western Pacific. He then did a residency in ophthalmology (eye surgery) at Naval Hospital Philadelphia. After becoming chief of the ophthalmology service at Naval Hospital Oakland, California, he returned to the School of Aviation Medicine in Pensacola, Florida, where he taught future flight surgeons. Following his retirement from the Navy in 1965, he trained residents at the Wills Eye Hospital in Philadelphia and then worked for the California State Department of Health as a medical consultant, retiring from that position in 1991. He lives in Tiburon, California.

JOHN FENWICK, after a long hospitalization, was declared permanently disabled and discharged from the Marine Corps in 1954. Since that time, he has made a living as a long-haul trucker, salesman, and commercial diver. He currently lives in Milton, Delaware.

ROBERT FLEISCHAKER retired from the Navy as a captain after twenty years of service and then practiced thoracic surgery until retiring again in 1987. He makes his home in Oceanside, California.

GARRISON "GUNNY" GIGG retired from the Marine Corps after nearly twenty-one years of service. He then worked for General Dynamics in the development of the M60 and M1A1 battle tanks. He lives in Fairfield Glade, Tennessee.

PEARCE GROVE left active duty in 1952 and joined the Coast Guard Reserve before receiving a Navy Reserve commission. He retired after a total of twenty-five years of military service. As a civilian, he made a living as an author, editor, archivist, and director of academic, research, and military libraries. He lives in Williamsburg, Virginia.

HERMES GRILLO is professor of surgery at Harvard Medical School and visiting surgeon and chief of general thoracic surgery (emeritus), Massachusetts General Hospital, Boston, Massachusetts.

ROBERT HARVEY, after returning from Korea, was stationed at Naval Hospital St. Albans, New York, for ten months before being separated from the Navy. He returned to private practice in Buffalo, New York, and became a clinical professor at the State University of New York (SUNY) Medical School in Buffalo. He retired from practice in 1988 and now lives in Venice, Florida.

BOBBI HOVIS became the first Navy nurse to volunteer for Vietnam duty in 1963. During her tour, she witnessed the coup that overthrew the Ngo Dinh Diem regime. She retired in 1967 with just over twenty years of Navy service. She resides in Annapolis, Maryland, and is the author of *Station Hospital Saigon: A Navy Nurse in Vietnam, 1963–1964*.

LILLIAN KEIL ended her Korean duty as an Air Force captain. Her combined World War II and Korean service makes her one of the most decorated women in U.S. military history. She makes her home in Covina, California.

DONALD KENT completed his Korean tour in June 1952 and eventually retired from the Navy after twenty-one years of service. He lives in Stonington, Connecticut.

CHESTER LESSENDEN, after his discharge from the Navy in 1953, practiced dermatology in Topeka, Kansas, until his retirement in 1986. He died in 1999.

HENRY LITVIN practiced psychiatry for many years after he was discharged from the Navy. He is retired and lives in Jenkintown, Pennsylvania.

DONALD LYON returned from Korea in 1951 and made a living in the dental supply business. He retired in 1988 and now lives in Thousand Oaks, California.

AARON MODANSKY resigned from the Naval Reserve in 1953 following the war and returned to his family's wholesale lumber business in New York. He retired in 1990, moved to Delray Beach, Florida, and joined the Civil Air Patrol flying search and rescue missions as commanding officer of CAP's Boca Raton Senior Squadron. "At 78, I hung up my spikes. I figured it was time for me to go. I love to fly and I enjoyed every minute of it. Above all, I love to be alive to talk about it."

STAVROS MOUNGELIS retired from the Marine Corps as a captain after twenty-one years of service. He then worked as a defense contractor for naval aviation. He lives in North Potomac, Maryland.

RAY MURRAY, commanding officer of the 5th Marines, retired from the Marine Corps as a major general after thirty-three years of service. During the Korean War, he earned two Army Silver Stars and his second Navy Cross, the first awarded during World War II for his action at Saipan. He makes his home in Oceanside, California.

RUSSELL O'DAY retired from the Navy in 1967 after twenty years of service. He then worked another twenty-three years for Brinks Incorporated. He lives in Stockbridge, Georgia.

JOSEPH OWEN went into the marketing business after the war. He is the author of *Colder Than Hell: A Marine Rifle Company at Chosin Reservoir.* Now retired, he divides his year between New York and Florida.

BILLY PENN, following his discharge from the Navy in 1955, continued his education where he left off, earning a degree and then going on to medical school. He practiced as an obstetrician-gynecologist in Baton Rouge, Louisiana, for thirty-two years. Because of his experiences as a POW, he never wanted to see anything Chinese again, but in the intervening years he delivered many babies to Chinese mothers. "God really has a sense of humor," he says.

HERBERT RENNER served one year as a reservist and twenty-two years in the regular Navy. He lives in Ridgecrest, California. "The chaos of fighting," he recalls, "left many voids, but I remember treating a great many wounded and dying. I never got hit. I could outrun a speeding bullet, although my helmet and flak jacket were a mess from shell fragments and my clothing was shredded in places."

CLIFFORD ROOSA resigned from the Navy in 1953, completed his surgical residency at St. Joseph's Hospital in Denver, Colorado, and practiced in Denver until 1977. He then worked as a contract physician at the Kwajalein Army Hospital at the Army's

Missile Research Center. In 1984, he began practice at a hospital in Bull Shoals, Arkansas, and later worked for an organization that filled temporary positions with physicians. "I'm licensed in seventeen states and practiced in most of them from one day to six months. I've had a lot of fun."

JAMES SARTORELLI left the Marine Corps in 1953 and went into the construction business. He still makes his living as a carpenter in Gaastra, Michigan.

MORTON SILVER earned the Silver Star for his heroism at Chosin Reservoir. He died in 2001.

HOWARD SIRAK was discharged from the Navy in 1953. He became professor of cardiac surgery at Ohio State University Hospital, Columbus, Ohio, before assuming a residency in heart and chest surgery at New York's Columbia Presbyterian Hospital. He returned to Ohio State University as assistant professor of cardiothoracic surgery and was appointed to the university's board of trustees. He ultimately became chairman of the board before retiring in 1981. He lives in Columbus, Ohio.

DAN SKILES retired from the Navy after being fitted with arm and leg prostheses. He worked at a service station "pumping gas and doing lube work," before attending business school under the GI Bill. He has been a freight and traffic clerk, a weighmaster at a stone quarry, an employee of the Disabled American Veterans, and a restaurateur. He now works as a certified evidence technician at the Pinole, California Police Department, and is Commander of the Jesse Orchard Post No. 2798, Veterans of Foreign Wars of the U.S., Rodeo, California.

HARRY SMART got out of the Marines in 1956 and joined the San Antonio Police Department. He spent thirty-eight years with the City of San Antonio and retired in 1998.

GLEN SNOWDEN went back to work as a postman when he returned from Korea despite the fact that he was missing an arm. He says, "I could deliver the mail just as good with one arm as with two." He is now retired and lives in Houston, Texas.

DOROTHY VENVERLOH retired from the Navy in 1970 after twenty-three years of service. She lives in St. Louis, Missouri.

THOMAS WADDILL was released in "Operation Little Switch" along with Billy Penn in April 1953. He returned home, was discharged, and eventually became an FBI agent. He died in 1999.

USS *CONSOLATION* (AH-15), remained in Korean waters for several months after the truce, continuing to support UN forces and caring for Korean civilians until the spring of 1954. Following an overhaul, *Consolation* took part in the evacuation of North Vietnamese refugees and their transfer to South Vietnam in "Operation Passage to Freedom." She then sailed north to Korea and once again served UN forces until 1955 when she was placed out of commission in reserve and berthed at San Francisco.

In 1960, the Navy transferred *Consolation* to the People to People Health Foundation, sponsor of "Project Hope." Under her new name SS *Hope*, the vessel visited ports in Southeast Asia, Africa, the Caribbean, and South America, providing treatment and training native hospital personnel in advanced medical and public health procedures. In 1974, for financial reasons, "Project Hope" relinquished the ship and she was returned to the Navy just long enough to have her stricken from the Navy register and transferred to the Maritime Administration for disposal. The old hospital ship was sold to Andy International, Inc., of Brownsville, Texas, in 1975 and scrapped.

USS *HAVEN* (AH-12), following her four tours of duty in Korea, took part in "Operation Repatriation," a rescue mission that returned to France 721 survivors of the epic siege of Dien Bien Phu in Vietnam. From 1956 until the middle 1960s, *Haven* remained tied to a pier at the U.S. Naval Station, Terminal Island, California. With her deck machinery "mothballed" and the door to her engine room sealed, she served as a station hospital for active duty and retired military personnel in the Los Angeles-Long Beach area. In 1967, *Haven* was transferred to the Maritime Administration and anchored in mothballs with the National Defense Reserve Fleet at Suisun Bay, California. Under the Ship Exchange Act, the Maritime Administration traded the vessel to Union Carbide. The company then converted her into a chemical tanker by welding a 330-foot section amidships. Renamed SS *Clendenin*, and then SS *Alaskan*, the old veteran was finally broken up for scrap in 1987.

USS *REPOSE* (AH-16), after shuttling patients around the Far East during late 1953 and early 1954, was decommissioned later that year. For more than ten years, she lay at anchor in mothballs with the National Defense Reserve Fleet at Suisun Bay, California, until the Navy reactivated her in 1965 for another war, this time in Southeast Asia. After reconditioning, *Repose* was recommissioned at Hunter's Point Naval Shipyard before heading for Vietnam waters. In February 1966, the vessel began cruising offshore near the DMZ, providing medical support for I Corps operations. By 1970, the "Angel of the Orient" had witnessed 14,000 helicopter landings, admitted over 24,000 patients, and treated more than 9,000 battle casualties. She returned home in 1970 and was decommissioned. Stricken from the Navy register in 1974, the veteran of three wars was transferred to the Maritime Administration for disposal.

Small Arms That Did the Damage

North Korean and Chinese Armies

Most small arms employed by the North Korean and Chinese armies were of pre-World War II and World War II Soviet manufacture. Later in the war, the Chinese produced weapons patterned after Soviet models. The Chinese communists also inherited large quantities of Japanese weapons from the Soviets, who confiscated them in Manchuria at the end of the Second World World War. The Red Chinese also captured American and British arms seized from the Nationalists who were defeated in the Chinese civil war.

Rifles, carbines, and automatic weapons

Mosin-Nagant (Russian [1891] and Soviet) bolt action rifles and carbines 7.62mm
Tokarev (Soviet) semi-automatic rifle 7.62mm
Type 38 bolt action rifle and carbine (Japanese) 6.5mm
Type 99 bolt action rifle (Japanese) 7.7mm
Antitank rifle (Russian) 14.5mm
PPSh-41 submachine gun "burp gun" (Soviet and Chinese) 7.62mm
World War II submachine guns (Japanese)
Type 50 submachine gun (Chinese) 7.62mm
Sten submachine gun (British) 9mm
Ruchnoy Pulemyot light machine gun (Russian) 7.62mm
Model 1910 Sokolov Pulemyot Maxima [Maxim type] (Russian) 7.62mm
Type 24 heavy machine gun (Chinese) 7.92mm

Grenades

Offensive or concussion (stick grenades based on Soviet RGD 33)
Fragmentation (based on Soviet RGD 33)

United Nations Forces

Most small arms used by United Nations forces were of U.S. and British manufacture and, with only slight modification, were of World War II vintage. Some weapons were of World War I or post-World War I design. The British Lee-Enfield rifle was of a pre-World War I design.

Rifles, carbines, and automatic weapons

M03A4 bolt action sniper rifle (U.S.) .30
M1 Garand rifle (U.S.) semi-automatic .30
M1C Garand (U.S.) sniper rifle .30
M1D Garand (U.S.) sniper rifle .30
M1 carbine (U.S.) semi-automatic .30
M2 carbine (U.S.) semi-automatic/automatic .30
M3 carbine (U.S.) semi-automatic/automatic .30
Browning Automatic Rifle [BAR] (U.S.) .30
M3A1 submachine gun "grease gun" (U.S.) .45
Thompson submachine gun (U.S.) .45
Lee-Enfield rifle (British) .303
Bren Mark IV light machine gun (British) .303
M1919A4 light machine gun (U.S.) .30

Grenades

Offensive or concussion (Mark I and Mark IIIA-1)
Fragmentation (Mark IIA1)

Glossary

Anastomosis: Removing a damaged portion of an artery or intestine and reattaching the vessel or organ end to end.

Aureomycin: Trademark for preparations of chlortetracycline hydrochloride used as an antibacterial and antiprotozoan.

Autoclave: An apparatus employing steam and pressure for sterilizing.

Barosinusitis: A condition produced by a difference between the atmospheric pressure of the environment and the air pressure in the paranasal sinuses.

Barotitis: A condition of the ear produced by exposure to differing atmospheric pressures.

Benzalkonium chloride: A water-soluble mixture of ammonium chloride derivatives, occurring as an amorphous powder or in gelatinous lumps. Used as an antiseptic and disinfectant.

Benzoin: A balsamic resin with an aromatic odor and taste used as a topical protectant.

Blakemore tube: A cannula made of the alloy vitallium and developed by Arthur H. Blakemore. Used to bridge arterial defects.

Bleeder: Any large blood vessel cut during a surgical procedure.

Cannula: A tube for insertion into a duct, cavity, or blood vessel.

Catgut: A sterile, absorbable suture material obtained from collagen of healthy mammals. Originally prepared from the submucous layer of sheep intestine.

Catheter: A tubular, flexible, surgical instrument for withdrawing fluids from (or introducing fluids into) a cavity of the body, especially one for introduction into the bladder through the urethra for the withdrawal of urine.

Carpule: A glass tube usually containing a premeasured dose of anesthetic.

Cauterization: The destruction of tissue with a hot iron, electric current, or a caustic substance such as phenol.

Chloramphenicol: An antibiotic substance originally derived from cultures of *Streptomyces venezuelae* and later produced synthetically. Used as an antibacterial and antirickettsial.

Chloromycetin: Trademark for preparations of chloramphenicol.

Chloroquine: A compound occurring as a white, or slightly yellow, crystalline powder with a bitter taste and soluble in water. Used as an antimalarial.

Chlortetracycline: See Aureomycin.

Clonazepam: A compound (benzodiazepine) used as an anticonvulsant and in the treatment of panic disorder.

Colostomy: The surgical creation of an opening between the colon and the surface of the body.

Debridement: The surgical removal of foreign material and dead or contaminated tissue from or adjacent to a wound until surrounding healthy tissue is exposed.

Demerol: Trademark for meperidine (pethidine) hydrochloride. A white, odorless powder soluble in water and alcohol used as a synthetic narcotic analgesic.

Dramamine: Trademark for preparations of dimenhydrinate, a white, odorless, crystallinepowder soluble in alcohol and chloroform used as an antinauseant.

Dysentery: An infectious disease marked by inflammation and ulceration of the lower part of the intestines. Characterized by chronic diarrhea and severe dehydration.

Edema: A swelling caused by abnormally large amounts of fluid in the subcutaneous tissues.

Epidemic hemorrhagic fever: An acute infectious disease characterized by fever, peripheral vascular collapse, and acute renal failure.

Excision: Removal of a growth or organ by cutting.

Fascia: A sheet or band of connective tissue surrounding, supporting, or binding together internal organs or parts of the body.

Frostbite: Damage to tissues resulting from exposure to low temperatures. Superficial frostbite may involve only the skin or extend to tissue immediately beneath it. Deep frostbite, resulting from extremely low temperatures, may affect not only the skin and subcutaneous tissue but also deeper tissues, sometimes leading to gangrene and loss of affected parts.

Gangrene: Death of large amounts of tissue due to an interruption of circulation followed by invasion of bacteria and putrefaction.

Guillotine amputation: The rapid amputation of a limb by a circular movement of the scalpel and then cut of the saw. The entire cross-section is left open for dressing. This procedure is performed when primary closure of the stump is contraindicated because of the possibility of recurrent or developing infection.

Hemoglobin: The oxygen-carrying pigment of red blood cells.

Hemostat: A small surgical clamp for constricting a blood vessel. Sometimes used as a locking plier for gripping a suture needle or surgical blade.

Heparin: An anticoagulant used in the prevention and treatment of thrombosis and in the repair of vascular injuries.

Induction: The production of anesthesia or unconsciousness by use of appropriate agents.

Laparoscope: A slender, illuminated optical or fiber-optic instrument that is inserted through an incision in the abdominal wall and used to examine visually the interior of the peritoneal cavity.

Laparoscopy: Examination of the interior of the abdomen by means of a laparoscope.

Laparotomy: A surgical incision into the abdominal cavity through any point in the abdominal wall.

Levin tube: A gastroduodenal catheter of sufficiently small caliber to permit transnasal passage.

Lidocaine: A white or yellow crystalline powder soluble in alcohol and chloroform used as a topical anesthetic.

Ligation: The application of any substance such as catgut, cotton, silk, or wire used to tie a vessel or strangulate a part.

MASH (Mobile Army Surgical Hospital): A mobile, multiple-bed hospital equipped for surgery and organized with personnel, equipment, and vehicles designed to operate close to tactical units.

Mercurochrome: Trademark for preparations of merbromin, a topical antibacterial.

Merthiolate: A water-soluble powder used as an antiseptic.

Metaphen: Trademark for preparations of nitromersol, a compound used topically in solution or tincture as a local anti-infective.

Morphine: An opium derivative used as a narcotic painkiller.

Nasogastric tube: A tube inserted into the nose and down the throat through which nourishment can be administered.

Nembutal: Trademark for preparations of sodium pentobarbital. A hypnotic used as a sedative, anticonvulsant, preanesthetic in surgery, or an adjunct to anesthesia.

Nitrous oxide: A colorless gas, N_2O, used as a general anesthetic or analgesic. Also called laughing gas.

Novocain: Trademark for procaine hydrochloride used as a local anesthetic.

Pediculi: Lice.

Penicillin: The so-called miracle antibiotic of World War II. Noted for its antibiotic properties by Sir Alexander Fleming in 1928, penicillin was first isolated from the penicillium mold in 1940. In the next several years, U.S. pharmaceutical firms began producing penicillin in quantities that made a huge impact in the treatment of Allied casualties during World War II. In common usage during the Korean War.

Perineum: The space between the anus and scrotum.

Periosteum: A specialized connective tissue covering all bones of the body and possessing bone-forming potential.

Peritoneum: The strong colorless membrane that lines the abdominopelvic walls and surrounds the viscera.

Peritonitis: Inflammation of the peritoneum accompanied by exudations of serum, fibrin, cells, and pus.

Plasma: The liquid part of blood, as distinguished from the suspended elements, such as platelets and red blood cells. Before serum albumin and whole blood were available, plasma was commonly used as a blood volume expander for the prevention and treatment of shock.

Popliteal: Pertaining to the posterior surface of the knee.

Primaquine: An orange-red, odorless crystalline powder (primaquine phosphate) with a bitter taste used to eliminate liver stages of *P.vivax* or *P.ovale* malaria.

Saphenous vein: Pertaining to or associated with a saphena, either of two large superficial veins of the leg.

Serum albumin: The principal protein of blood plasma. When administered intravenously, albumin draws fluid from surrounding tissues and helps increase blood volume to counteract shock.

Shock: A collapse of circulatory function caused by severe injury, blood loss, or disease and characterized by pallor, sweating, weak pulse, and very low blood pressure.

Smallpox: Variola; an acute infectious disease caused by a poxvirus.

Sodium pentothal: A commonly used anesthetic administered intravenously to induce general anesthesia.

Spica cast: A figure-of-8 cast with turns that cross one another at the shoulder or hip.

Stilette: A wire run through a catheter or cannula to render it stiff.

Stokes stretcher: A wire mesh and wood slat litter invented by Navy physician Charles F. Stokes. Stokes served as Surgeon General of the Navy from 1910 to 1914.

Streptomycin: A bactericidal antibiotic used chiefly in the treatment of tuberculosis.

Stryker frame: A rigid structure consisting of canvas stretched on anterior and posterior frames on which the patient can be rotated around his/her longitudinal axis. Commonly used in treating patients with broken backs.

Succinylcholine chloride: A white, odorless crystalline soluble in water, alcohol, and chloroform used as a skeletal muscle relaxant.

Sulfa drugs: A group of antibacterial compounds first introduced in 1936 to prevent or treat infection before penicillin came into general use in the mid-1940s. The World War II sulfa quintet included sulfanilamide, sulfapyridine, sulfathiazole, sulfadiazine, and sulfaguanidine.

Syrette: A single-dose, collapsible tube with an attached sterilized hypodermic needle sealed in tinfoil.

Terramycin: Trademark for preparations of oxytetracycline used as an antibacterial and antirickettsial.

Tetanus: An infectious, often fatal, disease caused by the toxic effect of *Clostridium tetani*. The bacteria usually enters the body through wounds. Characterized by violent muscle spasms, rigidity resulting in trismus (lockjaw), and respiratory failure.

Through-and-through wound: A continuous wound channel caused by a bullet or fragment that has entered and exited tissue.

Traction: The act of drawing or exerting a pulling force used principally in the treatment of fractures.

Triage: The sorting and classification of casualties to determine priority of need and proper place of treatment.

Urticaria: A vascular reaction of the skin marked by the transient appearance of smooth, slightly elevated patches (wheals), which are redder or paler than the surrounding skin and often attended by severe itching.

Vascular graft: The reconstruction of a damaged vessel by splicing in a section of vein.

Viscus: Any large interior organ in any one of the three great cavities of the body, especially in the abdomen. *Viscera* is the plural form.

Xylocaine: Trademark for preparations of lidocaine.

Bibliography

Published Sources

Apel, Otto F. Jr., and Apel, Pat. *MASH: An Army Surgeon in Korea.* Lexington, KY: The University Press of Kentucky, 1998.

Blair, Clay. *The Forgotten War: America in Korea 1950–1953.* New York: Times Books, 1987.

Blakemore, Arthur H., and Lord, Jere W. "A Nonsuture Method of Blood Vessel Anastomosis." *Journal of the American Medical Association* 127 (1945), 685–691.

Bridgman, Leonard. ed. and comp. *Jane's All the World's Aircraft.* London: Sampson Low, Marston and Co., Ltd., 1951–1952, 1952–1953, 1953–1954.

Chinnery, Philip D. *Korean Atrocity!: Forgotten War Crimes 1950–1953.* Annapolis: Naval Institute Press, 2000.

"Consolation." *Leatherneck* 35, no. 9, September 1952, 32–35.

Crosby, Nancy J. *Journal* (January 1952–September 1953), Nancy J. Crosby Collection, Arlington, VA: Women in Military Service for America Memorial Foundation, Inc.

Driscoll, Robert. "U.S. Army Helicopters in the Korean War." *Military Medicine* April 2001, 290–296.

Gablehouse, Charles. *Helicopters and Autogiros: A History of Rotating-Wing and V/STOL Aviation.* Philadelphia: J.B. Lippincott Company, 1969.

Haget, Carl. "Wound Ballistics and Body Armor in Korea," in *Wound Ballistics*, ed. John Coates (Washington: Office of the Surgeon General, Dept. of the Army, 1962), 691–768.

Harris, John F. "Practice of Field Medicine on Operation 'Killer.'" *The Military Surgeon* 109, no. 6, 683–688.

Hastings, Max. *The Korean War.* New York: Simon & Schuster, 1987.

Hering, Eugene R. "Combat Medical Practice." *The Military Surgeon, Journal of the Association of Military Surgeons of the United States.* Ed. James M. Phalen 110, January–June 1952. Washington: Association of Military Surgeons, United States. 1952, 102–106.

Hickey, Michael. *The Korean War: The West Confronts Communism.* Woodstock, NY: The Overlook Press, 2000.

The History of the Medical Department of the United States Navy, 1945–1955. NAVMED P-5057. Washington, DC: Bureau of Medicine and Surgery, 1955.

Holmes, Robert H., Enos, William F., Jr., and Beyer, James C. "Medical Aspects of Body Armor Used in Korea." *Journal of the American Medical Association* 155, no. 17, 1477–1478.

Massman, Emory A. *Hospital Ships of World War II: An Illustrated Reference to 39 United States Military Vessels.* Jefferson, NC: McFarland and Company, Inc., 1999.

Matray, James I., ed. *Historical Dictionary of the Korean War*, Greenwood Publishing Group, Westport, CT, 1991.

Omori, Frances. *Quiet Heroes: Navy Nurses of the Korean War 1950–1953: Far East Command.* St. Paul, MN: Smith House Press, 2000.

Owen, Joseph R. *Colder Than Hell: A Marine Rifle Company at Chosin Reservoir.* Annapolis: Naval Institute Press, 2000.

Russ, Martin. *Breakout: The Chosin Reservoir Campaign.* New York: Penguin Books, 1999.

San Francisco Daily News, 26 August 1950.

San Mateo [California] *Times*, 26 August 1950.

Smith, Joseph E. *Small Arms of the World.* Harrisburg, PA: Stackpole Books 1973.

Stokesbury, James L. *A Short History of the Korean War.* New York: William Morrow and Company, Inc., 1988.

Toland, John. *In Mortal Combat: Korea, 1950–1953.* New York: William Morrow and Company, Inc., 1991.

Weintraub, Stanley. *War in the Wards: Korea's Unknown Battle in a Prisoner-of-War Hospital Camp.* San Rafael, CA: Presidio Press, 1976.

Unpublished Sources

Boone, Joel T. *Joel T. Boone Papers: Memoirs* (unpublished), Washington, DC: Library of Congress, Ch. XXXVII, pp.171–180, Box 60. Courtesy of Milton F. Heller, Jr.

BUMED Archives, Washington. Medical Department Log, Headquarters, 1st Marine Division FMF, 14 July 1950–26 October 1950.

BUMED Archives, Washington Report of the U.S. Coast Guard Board of Inquiry into Sinking of USS *Benevolence*, 11 January 1951. *Benevolence* File.

BUMED Archives, Washington. Special Action Report: From E.A. Craig, commanding general, 1st Provisional Marine Brigade, FMF (Reinforced) to Commandant of the Marine Corps, Annex T, Report of Medical Section, 12 September 1950.

BUMED Archives, Washington. Special Action Report for period 28 August 1950 to 7 October 1950: 1st Marine Division, Annex "Queen," from Division Surgeon, Capt. Eugene Hering, MC, USN to Commanding General, 1st Marine Division, FMF.

BUMED Archives, Washington. USS *Haven* File.

Harrington, Eleanor. "Man Your Stations," manuscript in BUMED Archives.

Lessenden, Edith. Letter to author, 10 July 2001.

Medical Department, U.S. Navy. *Analysis of Problems Created by Korean Situation June 1950–March 1952.* Korea File, BUMED Archives, Washington.

Penn, Billy R. Reminsicences dated March 1995.

Venverloh, Dorothy. Letter dated September, 1950.

Waddill, Thomas H. Letter dated 26 March 1953.

First-Person Accounts
"Snafu Operation," from reminiscences of Chester M. Lessenden, Jr. (undated), and letter dated 13 August 1950.

"Culture Shock," adapted from a telephone interview by Jan K. Herman with Pearce S. Grove, 26 December 2000.

Chapter 2, "From Inchon to Seoul," adapted from telephone interviews by Jan K. Herman with Bill Davis, 17 April 2001; Donald Lyon, 27 December 2000; Robert J. Fleischaker, 11 January 2001; reminiscence of Chester M. Lessenden Jr., (undated); Henry Litvin, 15 June 2000; memoir of Joel T. Boone; Ray Murray, 9 July 2001; Russell O'Day, 24 July 2000; Garrison O. Gigg, 19 July 2000.

"First Encounter," adapted from a telephone interview by Jan K. Herman with Bill Davis, 17 April 2001.

"Cold Weather Combat," adapted from a telephone interview by Jan K. Herman with Garrison O. Gigg, 19 July 2000.

"Frozen in Memory," adapted from an interview by Jan K. Herman and David Lane with Henry Litvin, Jenkintown, PA, 21 June 2000.

"Bitter Cold and No Fires," from a letter of Chester M. Lessenden Jr., 11 or 12 December 1950.

"Silver Star Dentist," adapted from a telephone interview by Jan K. Herman with Morton Silver, 12 October 2000.

"Corpsman Down," adapted from a telephone interview by Jan K. Herman with Bill Davis, 17 April 2001.

"Circling the Wagons," adapted from an interview by Jan K. Herman with Joseph R. Owen, Washington, DC, 15 August, 2000.

"Flight Nurse Under Fire," adapted from a telephone interview by Jan K. Herman with Lillian Keil, 2 January 2001.

"Temporary Additional Duty," adapted from reminiscences of Robert P. Dobbie, 1994.

"Ward Victor," adapted from an interview by Jan K. Herman with Marilyn Ewing , Woodbridge, VA, 30 July 2001.

"No Fear of Flying," adapted from an interview by Jan K. Herman with Bobbi Hovis, Annapolis, MD, 2 December 1994.

"Unlucky AH-13," adapted from a telephone interview by Jan K. Herman with Dorothy J. Venverloh, 23 August 2000.

"Man Your Stations," from a manuscript of Eleanor Harrington for publication in the *American Journal of Nursing*.

"Angel of the Orient," adapted from an interview by Jan K. Herman with Lura Jane Emery, Annapolis, MD, 15 November 2001.

"*Haven* Anesthesiologist," adapted from a telephone interview by Jan K. Herman with Robert C. Harvey, 5 March 2001.

"To Have a Purpose," from journal of Nancy J. Crosby, January 1952–September 1953.

"Birth of the Helo Deck," from memoir of Joel T. Boone.

"First Helo Landing," adapted from a telephone interview by Jan K. Herman with Pearce S. Grove, 26 December 2000.

"Like a Hen on Her Eggs," from *Leatherneck*, September 1952.

"Cavalry from the Sky," adapted from a telephone interview by Jan K. Herman with Stavros S. Moungelis, 24 July 2000.

"Like a Bad Movie," adapted from a telephone interview by Jan K. Herman with Clifford Roosa, 13 December 2001.

"Flight Surgeon," adapted from a telephone interview by Jan K. Herman with Wayne Erdbrink, 23 September 2002.

"Pilot in Distress," adapted from a telephone interview by Jan K. Herman with Aaron Modansky, 18 September 2002.

"Surgical Team Eight," from reminiscences of Robert P. Dobbie, 1994.

"The Bunker War," adapted from a telephone interview by Jan K. Herman with Herbert G. Renner Jr., 10 April 2001.

"Catching Flak," adapted from a telephone interview by Jan K. Herman with James Sartorelli, 8 January 2002.

"Don't Let Me Die," adapted from a telephone interview by Jan K. Herman with Howard Sirak, 17 January 2001.

"Mini-MASH," from reminiscences of Howard S. Browne, (undated).

"Acting Battalion Surgeon," adapted from a telephone interview by Jan K. Herman with Donald C. Kent, 1 September 2000.

"This Was Not M*A*S*H," adapted from a telephone interview by Jan K. Herman with Hermes Grillo, 1 July 1999.

"The Smell of Cordite," adapted from a telephone interview by Jan K. Herman with Peter Bingheimer, 1 July 2002.

"All I Wanted Was a Chance," adapted from a telephone interview by Jan K. Herman with Dan Skiles, 2 and 7 May 2002.

"Nurse Amputee," adapted from a telephone interview by Jan K. Herman with Sarah Griffin Chapman, 18 March 2002.

"If They Can Do It, Why Can't I?" adapted from a telephone interview by Jan K. Herman with Rosella Nesgis Asbelle, 13 June 2002.

"'Bing' Crosby," adapted from a telephone interview by Jan K. Herman with Harry C. Smart, 26 December 2001.

"Bing's Story," adapted from a telephone interview by Jan K. Herman with Nancy J. Crosby, 26 December 2001.

"Marines and Rescuers," adapted from telephone interviews by Jan K. Herman with John L. Fenwick Jr., 25 October 2000; Glen C. Snowden, 26 October 2000; Richard Baiocchi, 28 June 2001; and Howard Sirak, 17 January 2001.

Index

British 101, 124, 215, 216
Chinese 2, 29, 39, 40, 41, 42, 44, 45, 47, 48, 49, 50, 51, 52, 56, 57, 58, 59, 62, 63, 68, 70, 76, 82, 103, 107, 111, 135, 136, 137, 138, 140, 141, 145, 146, 152, 162, 173, 175, 176, 177, 178, 179, 180, 182, 183, 184, 193, 211, 215
Coast Guard 93, 94, 210, 222
North Korean 1, 7, 8, 11, 14, 70, 101, 114, 125, 135, 155, 157, 162, 196, 205, 215
South Korean 19, 114, 123, 124, 144, 180, 193, 206, 207
Turks 101
U.S. 11, 18, 73, 93, 97, 99, 125, 128, 138, 167, 170, 206, 209, 211, 212, 213, 215, 216, 219, 221, 222
UN 3, 5, 14, 15, 19, 39, 101, 107, 108, 109, 111, 112, 114, 126, 128, 135, 138, 152, 182, 205, 212
United Nations 5, 39, 87, 98, 125, 215
Peters, Uel 25, 51
Pino, Dan 166, 168
Plasma 13, 17, 24, 33, 35, 64, 100, 152, 161, 162, 181, 186, 199, 201, 219, 220
POWs. *See* Prisoners of War
Prisoners of War 108, 173, 178
  American POWs 123
  Cuban POWs 179
  North Korean POWs 101
  POWs 101, 102, 123, 175, 179, 180
  South Korean POWs 123
Public Law 779 1
Punchbowl 138, 156, 161, 162, 167
Purple Heart 32, 33, 57, 74, 195
Pusan 3, 11, 12, 13, 14, 15, 16, 17, 19, 20, 21, 87, 96, 98, 101, 102, 106, 107, 108, 109, 110, 112, 120, 128, 155, 158, 161, 167

R

Red Beach 23, 26
Renner, Herbert G. 70, 138, 224
Rhee, Syngman 108, 110
Riggs, Cecil 90

Rochester, USS (CA-124) 27, 114, 115, 116, 117, 125
Roise, Harold 26, 34
Roosa, Clifford 6, 125, 126, 205, 224

S

Sartorelli 147, 224
Sartorelli, James 147, 212, 224
Scheddel, Thomas A. 173
Seasickness 12, 126
Seoul 2, 7, 21, 27, 28, 29, 30, 31, 32, 33, 34, 35, 36, 39, 45, 56, 68, 110, 121, 123, 124, 135, 136, 158, 175, 182, 206, 207, 223
Seydel, Karle 51, 52
Sherman, Forrest 94
Shimonoseki Straits 104, 107
Shoemaker, Robert 155
Silver, Morton I. 30
Silver, Morton Israel 6, 55, 56, 57, 212
Silver Star 30, 55, 58, 198, 212, 223
Sirak, Howard 151, 152, 199, 203, 204, 224
Skiles, Dan 7, 8, 185, 190, 212, 224
Smart, Harry 192, 195, 196, 207, 212, 224
Snowden, Glen 8, 197, 198, 201, 202, 212, 224
Sodium pentothal 104, 153, 220
Sokcho-ri 118
Soyanggang River 152
St. Paul, USS (CA-73) 126, 127, 205, 222
Stelter, Frederick 127
Stevenson, C.A. "Red" 157
Struble, Arthur D. 115, 117, 118
Succinylcholine chloride 104, 220
Sudong 39, 40, 41, 44
Sulfa 3, 23, 35, 41, 47, 49, 154, 220
Sun Shipbuilding and Dry Dock Company 94
Swanson, Clifford 190

T

Taegu 156, 158
Tarr, George 168
TB. *See* tuberculosis
Terramycin 3, 154, 220

Printed in the United States
94606LV00003B/49/A